Lecture Notes on
Clinical Pharmacology

Lecture Notes on Clinical Pharmacology

JOHN L. REID
DM FRCP
Regius Professor of Materia Medica

PETER C. RUBIN
DM MRCP
Senior Registrar in Clinical Pharmacology

BRIAN WHITING
MD FRCP
Senior Lecturer in Clinical Pharmacology

Department of Materia Medica
University of Glasgow

BLACKWELL SCIENTIFIC PUBLICATIONS
OXFORD LONDON EDINBURGH
BOSTON MELBOURNE

© 1982 by
Blackwell Scientific Publications
Editorial offices:
Osney Mead, Oxford, OX2 0EL
8 John Street, London, WC1N 2ES
9 Forrest Road, Edinburgh, EH1 2QH
52 Beacon Street, Boston
  Massachusetts 02108, USA
99 Barry Street, Carlton,
  Victoria 3053, Australia

First published 1982

Typeset
by Santype International Ltd.,
Salisbury, and printed and bound by
Billing and Sons Limited, London,
Oxford, Worcester.

DISTRIBUTORS

USA
  Blackwell Mosby Book
  Distributors
  11830 Westline Industrial Drive
  St. Louis, Missouri 63141

Canada
  Blackwell Mosby Book
  Distributors
  120 Melford Drive, Scarborough
  Ontario, M1B 2X4

Australia
  Blackwell Scientific Book
  Distributors
  214 Berkeley Street, Carlton
  Victoria 3053

British Library
Cataloguing in Publication Data

Reid, John L.
  Lecture notes on clinical pharma-
    cology.
  1. Pharmacology
  I. Title   II. Rubin, Peter C.
  III. Whiting, Brian
  615'.1   RM300

  ISBN 0-632-00896-2

Contents

Preface

Clinical pharmacology is a new and rapidly expanding specialty which has grown in importance with the increase in both the number and the complexity of drugs. Bridging the gap between laboratory science and the practice of medicine at the bedside, clinical pharmacology has as its primary aim the promotion of safe and effective drug use: to optimise benefits and minimise risks.

Developments in medicine, pharmacology and physiology have led to a better understanding of disease processes and a more rational use of drugs. Recent years have seen the development of drugs designed to interact with specific receptors or enzyme systems. In addition the application of biochemical and immunological techniques has led to a clearer appreciation of the mechanisms involved in adverse drug reactions and interactions. With this understanding has come the potential to reduce greatly the number of unwanted drug effects. The intensity of drug action is often related to plasma concentration, and recent advances in analytical techniques have enabled rapid and accurate determination of the plasma concentrations of many drugs. This provides an added dimension to the optimisation of drug use.

For many years we have taught clinical pharmacology to medical practitioners and undergraduate students. We have now been persuaded by our students that there is a need for a brief, clearly written and up to date review of clinical pharmacology. *Lecture Notes on Clinical Pharmacology* has been prepared to meet this need. We have not attempted to be comprehensive, but have tried to emphasise the principles of clinical pharmacology, areas which are developing rapidly and topics which are of particular clinical importance. The book is based on the four term course of

vii

lectures and seminars in clinical pharmacology and therapeutics for medical students at the University of Glasgow. In addition, we have drawn on our experience of organising courses for postgraduate students, general practitioners and medical specialists. Thus, while intended primarily for medical students, we believe this book will also be of use to those preparing for higher examinations and doctors in established practice who wish to remain well informed of current concepts in clinical pharmacology.

For all who use it, we hope this book will provide a clear understanding not only of *how* but also of *when* to use drugs.

John Reid
Peter Rubin
Glasgow, December 1981   Brian Whiting

Acknowledgements

We have been fortunate in obtaining the assistance of many colleagues in Glasgow during the preparation of this volume. In particular, we would like to acknowledge the contributions of those who participate in the undergraduate teaching programme in clinical pharmacology and who contributed to the writing, preparation, revision and editing of several chapters: Dr George Addis, Dr Alistair Beattie, Mr Scott Bryson, Dr Brian Campbell, Professor Kenneth Calman, Dr Henry Elliott, Dr William Fulton, Dr Stewart Hillis, Professor David Lawson, Dr Walter Nimmo.

We are very grateful to several colleagues who have given their time to provide valuable criticism of chapters relating to their special interest: Dr Ian Bone, Dr Brooke Hogg, Dr Fiona Logan, Dr Nancy Loudon, Dr Hamish McLaren, Dr Paul McGill, Mr Paul O'Donnell.

We owe a great debt of gratitude to Mrs Mary Wood and Miss Eleanor Newell for their considerable efforts in typing and collating the material over a very short time and thank the other secretaries in the department for their invaluable assistance. The Audiovisual Department at Stobhill Hospital kindly assisted with the artwork. We greatly appreciate the work of Miss Randa Pharaon who performed a substantial task in sub-editing the manuscript before submission to the publishers. We thank Dr Michael Orme, Reader in Clinical Pharmacology at the University of Liverpool for his constructive review of the text. Mr Per Saugman and Mr Robert Campbell of Blackwell Scientific Publications have advised, guided and encouraged us throughout and to them also we offer our thanks.

We ourselves accept full responsibility for the contents of the volume and for any mistakes or misunderstandings.

John Reid
Peter Rubin
Brian Whiting

Principles of clinical pharmacology

Until the twentieth century, medical practice depended largely on the administration of mixtures of natural plant or animal substances. These preparations contained a number of pharmacologically active agents in variable amounts. Their actions and indications were empirical and based on historical or traditional experience. Their use was rarely based on an understanding of the mechanism of disease or careful critical measurement of effect.

During the last 80 years, an increased understanding of biochemical and pathophysiological factors in disease has developed. The chemical synthesis of agents with well characterised, specific actions on cellular mechanisms has led to the introduction of many powerful and effective drugs.

1.1 PRINCIPLES OF DRUG ACTION

Application of drug treatment

Pharmacological agents are used in therapeutics to:
  (1) Cure disease:
    chemotherapy in cancer or leukaemia,
    antibiotics in specific bacterial infections.

1

(2) Alleviate symptoms:
antacids in dyspepsia,
non-steroidal anti-inflammatory drugs in rheumatoid arthritis.
(3) Replace deficiencies:
restoration of normal function by the replacement of a
deficiency in endogenous hormone, enzyme or transmitter.

A *drug* is a single chemical entity that may be one of the
constituents of a medicine.

A *medicine* may contain one or more active constituents (drugs)
together with additives to facilitate administration (colouring,
flavouring, and other excipients).

Mechanism of drug action

Drugs may act in several different ways and our understanding of
the mechanism of drug action advances hand-in-hand with
developments in basic and clinical science.

Action on a specific receptor

Receptors are macromolecular structures linked to effector mechanisms which interact with drugs to form a drug–receptor complex.
This interaction may be reversible or irreversible.

Agonist drugs stimulate or activate the receptor to produce an
effect. Antagonist drugs block the effects that usually result from
stimulation of the receptor by agonists. Antagonism is either *competitive* if the drug–receptor interaction is reversible, or *non-
competitive* if the drug–receptor complex is irreversible.

Blockade by a competitive antagonist *can be overcome* by large
amounts of agonist.

Competitive antagonism is generally of short duration and
depends on the presence of drug. For examples, Beta-receptor
antagonists, such as propranolol block the chronotropic and
inotropic effects of increased catecholamine release. Opiate receptor
antagonists, such as naloxone reverse the respiratory depressant
and sedative effects of morphine.

Non-competitive antagonism *is not reversed* by any amount of
agonist, is usually long-lasting (days or weeks) and may persist
after the drug has been withdrawn. Recovery depends on the
synthesis of new receptors.

For example, phenoxybenzamine, which irreversibly blocks alpha adrenoceptors.

Action on specific enzymes

Enzymes, like receptors, are protein macromolecules with which substrates interact to activate or inhibit enzymatic activity. Inhibition of enzyme activity may be *competitive* (reversible) and relatively short-lasting. For example allopurinol, a xanthine oxidase inhibitor and carbidopa a decarboxylase inhibitor.

Alternatively it may be *non-competitive* (irreversible) and long-lasting, persisting until new enzyme protein has been synthesised. For example, prostaglandin synthetase inhibitors such as aspirin, and monoamine oxidase inhibitors such as phenelzine.

Action on membranes

The electrophysiological processes that form the basis of nerve and muscle function depend on ion fluxes to alter transmembrane potential. Various drugs can influence these ionic movements:
 Antiarrhythmic drugs,
 Anticonvulsant drugs,
 General anaesthetics.

Cytotoxic actions

Drugs used in cancer or in the treatment of infections may kill malignant cells or micro-organisms. Often the mechanisms have been defined in terms of effects on specific receptors or enzymes. In other cases chemical action (alkylation) damages DNA or other macromolecules and results in cell death or failure of cell division.

1.2 PRINCIPLES OF DRUG ABSORPTION

Bioavailability

Some drugs are applied directly to their sites of action. Examples of such topical administration include the application of fungicides to

TABLE 1.1   Modes of drug administration

Parenteral	Enteral	Topical
Intravenous	Oral	Determatological
Intramuscular	Sublingual	Ocular
Subcutaneous	Rectal	Inhalational
Intrathecal		
Intra-articlar		

infected skin and steroid or bronchodilator aerosols in the treatment of asthma. However, in most cases a drug must be transported to its site of action by the systemic circulation.

Bioavailability is the term used to describe the *proportion of administered drug that reaches the systemic circulation in unchanged form.*

In the case of intravenous administration bioavailability will clearly be 100%, but most drugs are given orally and numerous factors can prevent complete absorption. Among the more important are the presence of food, the barrier presented by the lipid membranes of the gut and first-pass metabolism.

First-pass metabolism

First-pass or pre-systemic metabolism refers to *metabolism of a drug that occurs en route from the gut lumen to the systemic circulation.*

Some drugs, e.g. chlorpromazine and levodopa, are metabolised in the gut wall, but in most cases first-pass metabolism occurs in the liver. This is so complete with lignocaine and glyceryl trinitrate that bioavailability following oral administration is zero. However, drugs normally given orally can have extensive first-pass metabolism: e.g. propranolol is about 80% metabolised before it reaches the systemic circulation.

The importance of first-pass metabolism is twofold:

(1) It is a major reason for apparent differences in drug absorption between individuals. Even healthy people show considerable variation in liver metabolising capacity.

(2) In patients with severe liver disease, a far greater proportion of drugs that normally undergo extensive first-pass metabolism is absorbed *unchanged*. This is discussed in detail in Chapter 2.3.

1.3 PRINCIPLES OF DRUG DISTRIBUTION

Volume of distribution

Most drugs are not wholly confined to the blood but are distributed throughout the body to other tissues. Many factors determine the extent of distribution; the most important are:

The ability of a drug to cross lipid membranes. For example, drugs that are ionised at physiological pH tend to distribute poorly because ionisation tends to preclude passage across lipid membranes.

The extent of binding to plasma proteins. Drugs that are highly protein bound distribute less extensively than those with low binding.

A knowledge of the extent of drug distribution is important because:

(1) When a drug is extensively distributed outside the blood, it is not easily removed from the body by techniques such as haemodialysis, which remove drug from blood. For example, well over 95% of digoxin in the body is distributed outside the blood. Thus, if a person has taken an overdose of the drug there is no advantage in trying to speed elimination by dialysis.

(2) A drug that is distributed outside the circulation provides a reservoir from which the blood is continuously replenished as drug elimination from the body occurs. If this reservoir is large, i.e. distribution is extensive, fluctuations of drug concentration in blood are damped. In other words, swings from peak to trough concentration between doses are less dramatic than for drugs less widely distributed.

The extent of distribution is expressed in numerical terms as: *Apparent volume of distribution,* which is *the volume that would be occupied by the drug if all the drug in the body had the same concentration as the drug in blood.*

This is an *abstract* concept. Volumes of distribution often *far exceed* the total body volume because drug may be concentrated in certain tissues such as fat. However, it is useful to have a numerical means of describing the extent of distribution. Examples are shown in Table 1.2.

TABLE 1.2 Volumes of distribution of some commonly used drugs

Drug	Volume of distribution (litres/70 kg)
Nortriptyline	1200
Digoxin	600
Propranolol	250
Lignocaine	120
Phenytoin	40
Theophylline	25
Gentamicin	20
Warfarin	9
Tolbutamide	8

Protein binding

A proportion of any drug circulating in blood is usually attached by physicochemical forces to plasma proteins, and a proportion is free or unbound in solution. Only the unbound drug is available for pharmacological action at receptors. Protein binding becomes clinically important when it involves a high proportion, i.e. > 90% of drug in the blood. Drugs that are highly protein bound are listed in Table 1.3. One consequence of high protein binding is that it limits distribution of drug to other body tissues, as indicated above. A second consequence is that it limits the amount of free drug available for pharmacological effect, and clinically relevant effects may become apparent when the extent of binding is altered by:

Disease. Plasma proteins are altered both in quantity and chemical characteristics in renal and hepatic disease: there is a decrease in drug binding. This is discussed in Chapter 2.2 and 2.3.

TABLE 1.3 Drugs that are highly (> 90%) protein bound

Phenytoin	Frusemide
Tolbutamide	Warfarin
Diazoxide	Phenylbutazone
Propranolol	Chlorpromazine
Prazosin	Tricyclic antidepressants

Drugs competing for protein-binding sites. Theoretically competition for binding sites may result in an increase in the free concentration of one drug, but rapid redistribution and clearance of this fraction precludes the risk of toxicity.

The major plasma protein involved in drug binding has long been thought to be albumin. However, certain basic drugs also bind to alpha-1-acid glycoprotein, e.g. propranolol, prazosin and chlorpromazine. This is an acute phase protein whose concentration rises in acute inflammation with a resulting decrease in free-drug concentration. The clinical significance is uncertain.

1.4 PRINCIPLES OF DRUG ELIMINATION

Drug metabolism

Drugs are eliminated from the body by two principal mechanisms: (1) liver metabolism and, (2) renal excretion. Drugs that are already water soluble are generally excreted unchanged by the kidney. Lipid-soluble drugs are not easily excreted by the kidney because, following glomerular filtration, they are largely reabsorbed from the proximal tubule. The first step in the elimination of such lipid-soluble drugs is metabolism to more polar (water-soluble) compounds. This is achieved mainly in the liver, and generally occurs in two phases:

(1) Mainly oxidation (sometimes reduction or hydrolysis) to a more polar compound,

(2) Conjugation, usually with glucuronic or sulphuric acid.

Phase 1 metabolism

Oxidation can occur in various ways: hydroxylation, oxygenation at carbon, nitrogen or sulphur atoms, *N*- and *O*-dealkylation or deamination. These reactions are catalysed by the mixed function oxidases of the endoplasmic reticulum which comprise at least four types of enzymes: cytochrome P–450 and b5 with their corresponding reductases. The biochemistry of the mixed function oxidase system has not been fully elucidated. It is known, however, that there are multiple forms of cytochrome P–450, which can act on numerous substrates.

Phase 1 metabolites usually have only minor structural differences from the parent drug but may exhibit totally different pharmacological actions. For example, the aromatic hydroxylation of phenobarbitone abolishes its hypnotic activity, while metabolism of azathioprine produces the powerful antimetabolite 6-mercaptopurine.

Phase 2 reactions

These involve the addition of small endogenous molecules to the phase 1 metabolite, and almost always lead to abolition of pharmacological activity. Like phase 1 reactions, the liver is the major site but conjugation can occur in the gut wall where it can contribute to first-pass metabolism.

For most drugs, the rate of metabolism is directly proportional to the concentration of drug at the enzyme receptor site, and the concentration of drug in blood is proportional to the dose given. In these circumstances, elimination from the body is referred to as a first-order process. If the capacity of drug metabolising enzymes is exceeded, however, there is an accumulation of drug as elimination proceeds by a zero-order process. This implies that drug concentration in the blood increases out of proportion to increases in dose. Fortunately this occurs infrequently, the most important clinical example being the anticonvulsant phenytoin (p. 44). The enzymes that metabolise phenytoin can become saturated at therapeutic drug concentrations, and small increases in dose can produce large increases in phenytoin concentration. Therapeutic drug monitoring in these circumstances is vital (Chapter 5.1).

Metabolic drug interactions

The wide range of drugs metabolised by the mixed function oxidase system provides the opportunity for interactions of two types:

(1) *Induction*. Enzyme activity increases as the concentration of substrate increases. If two drugs which are metabolised by the same enzyme are given together, each can influence the metabolism of the other. For example, the anticonvulsants phenytoin, carbamazepine and phenobarbitone are all metabolised by the same enzymes that metabolise the constituents of oral contraceptives. If a woman receiving an oral contraceptive starts taking one of these

anticonvalsants, the metabolism of the oestrogen and progestagen in the oral conctraceptive increases with the risk of contraceptive failure. This phenomenon is not limited to drug administration. Cigarette smoking, for example, results in enzyme induction with increased metabolism of theophylline.

(2) *Inhibition.* Concurrently administered drugs can also lead to an inhibition of enzyme activity. Sulphonamides, for example, decrease the metabolism of phenytoin so that phenytoin blood levels become toxic. Similarly, cimetidine decreases the metabolism of propranolol, leading to enhanced bradycardia.

Genetic factors in metabolism

There are wide variations in the rate at which apparently similar healthy people metabolise drugs. Studies with monozygotic and dizygotic twins have shown this difference to have a strong genetic basis, although rather poorly defined environmental factors also make a contribution. There are a number of specific examples which are clinically important:

(1) Acetylation in the liver is under polymorphic genetic control, the activity of *N*-acetyltransferase being determined by a recessive gene. Approximately 50% of Caucasians are slow acetylators and the following drugs are known to be cleared from the body more slowly in such people: isoniazid, hydralazine, procainamide, sulphonamides and dapsone. Slow acetylators are more likely to develop concentration related adverse effects, e.g. the lupus erythematosus syndrome with hydralazine or procainamide. These patients should receive lower doses of drug than fast acetylators.

(2) Oxidation at a carbon atom also shows genetic polymorphism, but here the number of poor metabolisers is small: about 5% of the Caucasian population. Drugs that are known to be affected are nortriptyline, phenformin and debrisoquine. At least the last two drugs are very rarely used now because of adverse effects. In retrospect it seems likely that these problems were partly due to relatively poor metabolism in some individuals.

Renal excretion

Three processes are implicated in renal excretion of drugs:

(1) *Glomerular filtration.* This is the most common route of renal

elimination. The free drug is cleared by filtration, and the protein bound drug remains in the circulation where some dissociates to restore equilibrium.

(2) *Active secretion at the proximal tubule.* Both weak acids and weak bases have specific secretory sites in proximal tubular cells. Penicillins are eliminated by this route as is about 60% of procainamide.

(3) *Passive reabsorption in the distal tubule.* This occurs only with un-ionised, i.e. lipid-soluble, drugs. Whether or not weak acids and bases are reabsorbed depends on urine pH, which determines the degree of ionisation. This fact is utilised in enhancing the renal elimination of aspirin following an overdose (p. 314).

If renal function is impaired, for example by disease or old age, then there is a decrease in the elimination rate of drugs that usually undergo renal excretion (Chapter 2.2).

The rate at which drugs are eliminated is expressed in numerical terms as: *Clearance,* which is defined as *the volume of fluid that is completely cleared of drug in unit time.* It is usually expressed as ml/min or l/h. This is discussed further on p. 43.

Comment

The disposition or *pharmacokinetics* of a drug is determined by its absorption, distribution and elimination and depends on its physical and chemical properties. The effects or *pharmacodynamics* of a drug are determined by its action on specific receptors and the concentration of the drug at the receptor site.

CHAPTER 2

Influence of disease on pharmacokinetics and pharmacodynamics

Drugs are usually considered in terms of their effect on disease processes. However, several diseases can influence the pharmacokinetics of a drug or its pharmacodynamic effect on target organs. This is of considerable clinical importance when diseases of the liver or kidney modify drug elimination, or drug distribution and elimination are altered in congestive cardiac failure.

2.1 INFLUENCE OF GASTROINTESTINAL DISEASE

Achlorhydria

Aspirin and cephalexin are poorly absorbed. These drugs have an acid pKa and the *absence* of acid in the stomach favours ionisation of drug molecules, limiting absorption.

Coeliac disease

There are several pathophysiological factors that can influence drug absorption. In addition to the considerable loss of absorptive surface, the rate of gastric emptying is increased, intraluminal pH is increased, the enterohepatic circulation is decreased, permeability of the gut wall is increased, intestinal drug metabolism is decreased, and activity of various enzymes such as esterases is decreased. The outcome is complex and while some drugs show decreased absorption, e.g. amoxycillin and pivampicillin, others show increased absorption, e.g. cephalexin and co-trimoxazole, and some show no change, e.g. ampicillin.

Crohn's disease

Again there are several changes that can influence drug absorption. The absorptive surface area is decreased, the gut wall is thickened and bacterial flora is altered. The absorption of the two components of co-trimoxazole is affected in opposite ways: that of trimethoprim is decreased, while sulphamethoxazole absorption is increased.

Comment

Many factors can influence drug absorption when the gastrointestinal tract is abnormal. The presence of a malabsorption syndrome does not imply that drugs are necessarily malabsorbed: the absorption of some can actually increase. There is currently insufficient information to comment on the clinical importance of these changes, but theoretically, treatment failure may occur because of malabsorption, and drug toxicity may result from increased absorption.

2.2 INFLUENCE OF IMPAIRED RENAL FUNCTION

Impaired renal function can influence the following aspects of drug therapy:
  (1) Altered pharmacokinetics.
      (a) Decreased elimination of drugs that are normally excreted entirely or mainly by the kidneys.
      (b) Decreased protein binding.
  (2) Altered drug effect.
  (3) Worsening of existing clinical condition.

(4) Enhancement of drug adverse effects.

Each of these factors is now considered in more detail.

Altered pharmacokinetics

Elimination

Since the kidney represents one of the major routes of drug elimination, a decrease in normal function can influence the clearance of many drugs. If a drug normally cleared by the kidney is given to someone with decreased renal function without altering the dose, the blood concentration of that drug increases. The worse the renal function, the higher the concentration. This is of considerable importance in the case of drugs showing concentration related adverse effects, particularly those in which toxic effects occur just above the therapeutic range.

When drugs are given to patients with renal dysfunction, therefore, the aim is to achieve the same concentrations which are seen in patients with normal kidneys. This is done as follows:

(1) Determine renal function, either by measuring creatinine clearance (based on a 24 h urine collection) or by estimating creatinine clearance from the serum creatinine concentration.

(2) Modify dose, either by increasing the dosage interval or by giving less drug at the usual frequency.

In severe renal failure these two approaches are often combined: less drug is given less often than usual. The necessary extent and precision of dose modification depends very much on the toxicity of the drug concerned. In the case of aminoglycosides, even minor impairment of renal function requires some modification of dose while the dose of penicillins need only be reduced in *severe* renal failure (creatinine clearance < 10 ml/min). Guidance on dosage reduction is available for most commonly used drugs and nomograms exist for those with a high risk of toxicity.

(3) Give a loading dose. This is necessary if therapeutic concentrations have to be established rapidly, since about five half-lives are required to achieve steady-state drug concentrations: the prolonged half-life resulting from renal failure delays the attainment of steady state.

(4) Monitor drug concentrations. This is mandatory for drugs with serious concentration-related adverse effects, e.g. aminoglycosides and digoxin. Nomograms are useful guides to the

doses likely to be appropriate, but every patient is different. Measured concentrations of drugs in the blood must be used to assess the altered kinetics and to determine the most appropriate dose. This is discussed further in Chapter 5.1.

Decreased protein binding

The following changes occur in patients with impaired renal function:

(1) Acidic drugs are less bound but the binding of basic drugs undergoes little or no change.

(2) The decrease in binding is correlated with the severity of renal impairment.

(3) Haemodialysis does not return binding to normal but renal transplantation does.

(4) The structure of albumin is changed in renal failure and this probably explains in large part the changes in binding.

The clinical relevance of decreased protein binding is demonstrated by the interpretation of serum phenytoin concentrations in renal failure. The usually quoted therapeutic range of phenytoin is 10–20 μg/ml, which represents total (bound and unbound) drug. In renal failure the proportion of bound drug falls and free phenytoin concentration increases. This excess free phenytoin is largely eliminated by the liver, where the extent of phenytoin metabolism is proportional to free drug concentration. A new equilibrium is therefore established in renal failure where *bound* phenytoin is reduced but *free* phenytoin concentration is unchanged. Since it is the free phenytoin which is pharmacologically active, the concentration of phenytoin necessary to produce a therapeutic effect is reached at a lower *total* phenytoin concentration. Putting this in numerical terms, the therapeutic range for phenytoin in severe renal failure is 5–10 μg/ml.

Altered drug effect

Independent of changes in pharmacokinetics there are several examples of increased sensitivity to drug effects in renal failure. Opiates, barbiturates, phenothiazines and benzodiazepines all show greater central nervous system effects in patients with renal failure compared to those with normal renal function. The reason is not known, but meningeal permeability is increased in renal failure and this could be one explanation.

Various antihypertensive drugs have a greater postural effect in renal failure. Again the reasons are not clear but changes in sodium balance and autonomic dysfunction may be partly responsible.

Worsening of the existing clinical condition

Drug therapy can result in deterioration of the clinical condition in the following ways:

(1) *By further impairing renal function.* In patients with renal failure it is clearly desirable to avoid drugs that are known to be nephrotoxic and for which alternatives are available. Examples include cephaloridine, cephalothin, penicillamine and gold.

(2) *By causing fluid retention.* Fluid balance is a major problem in the more severe forms of renal failure. Drugs that cause fluid retention should therefore be avoided, e.g. carbenoxolone and anti-inflammatory drugs such as indomethacin.

(3) *By increasing the degree of uraemia.* Tetracyclines, except doxycycline, have an anti-anabolic effect and should be avoided.

Enhancement of drug adverse effects

(1) *Digoxin.* In addition to the decreased elimination referred to earlier, digoxin is more likely to cause adverse effects in patients with severe renal failure if there are substantial electrolyte abnormalities, particularly hypercalacaemia and/or hypokalaemia.

(2) *Potassium sparing diuretics.* Since potassium elimination is impaired in renal failure, diuretics which also conserve potassium (amiloride, spironolactone) are more likely to cause hyperkalaemia.

(3) *Lactic acidosis.* Phenformin, and probably to a lesser extent, metformin, are much more likely to produce lactic acidosis in patients with renal failure.

2.3 INFLUENCE OF LIVER DISEASE

Impaired liver function can influence the response to treatment in several ways:

(1) Altered pharmacokinetics
    (a) Increased bioavailability resulting from reduced first-pass metabolism.
    (b) Decreased protein binding.
    (c) Decreased elimination.
(2) Altered pharmacodynamics.
(3) Worsening of metabolic state.

Altered pharmacokinetics

The liver is the largest organ in the body, has a substantial blood supply (around 1.5 l/min) and is interposed between the gastrointestinal tract and the systemic circulation. For these reasons it is uniquely suited for the purpose of influencing drug metabolism.

Decreased first-pass metabolism

For the majority of drugs given orally, absorption occurs across that portion of the gastrointestinal epithelium that is drained by veins forming part of the hepatoportal system. Before reaching the systemic circulation such drugs must pass through the liver and are, therefore, exposed to enzymes in that organ which metabolise drugs. For drugs that are susceptible to such hepatic metabolism, a substantial proportion of an orally administered dose can be metabolised before it ever reaches its site of pharmacological action. This phenomenon is referred to as first-pass metabolism and has two major determinants: (1) hepatocellular function and (2) portosystemic shunting. A decrease in hepatocellular function decreases the capacity of the liver to perform metabolic processes, while portosystemic shunting directs drug away from sites of metabolism. Both factors are usually present in patients with severe cirrhosis. Drugs with a high first-pass metabolism are listed in Table 2.1.

TABLE 2.1   Drugs showing high first-pass metabolism

Aspirin, Chlormethiazole, Chlorpromazine, Labetalol, Lignocaine, Metoprolol, Morphine, Nitroglycerine, Nortriptyline, Paracetamol, Pentazocine, Pethidine, Prazosin, Propoxyphene and Propranolol.

Knowledge of the drugs that undergo first-pass metabolism is important in situations where it is decreased as the result of disease. Considerably more active drug then reaches the site of action and any given dose of drug has unexpectedly intense effects.

Examples for patients with severe cirrhosis are:
Chlormethiazole (bioavailability tenfold increase),
Labetalol (twofold increase),
Paracetamol (50% increase),
Pentazocine (fourfold increase),
Pethidine (twofold increase),
Propranolol (twofold increase).

Decreased protein binding

Decreased elimination by liver metabolism

These aspects are interdependent and should, therefore, be considered together.

In this context, drugs can be classified according to the ability of the liver to metabolise them.

Flow-limited drugs. These are drugs that the liver metabolises at a very high rate. Their clearance is dependent only on the rate at which drug is delivered to the enzyme systems and is proportional to blood flow. The clearance of these drugs is sensitive to factors which can influence hepatic blood flow.

Examples: Lignocaine, propranolol, pethidine, pentazocine, propoxyphene, nortriptyline and morphine.

Capacity-limited drugs. The rate of metabolism of drugs in this class is sufficiently low that hepatic clearance is not limited by the amount of drug delivered to the liver but is dependent on the capacity of the liver enzymes to metabolise the drugs concerned. The rate of metabolism of these drugs is dependent on the concentration of drug at the enzyme receptor site, which is proportional to the free concentration of drug in plasma. For this reason, the metabolism of these drugs can be further divided into protein binding sensitive and insensitive categories:

Capacity-limited, binding-sensitive drugs are those which are highly protein bound. Conditions that affect protein binding can thus have a significant effect on their hepatic clearance.

Examples include: Phentytoin, diazepam, tolbutamide, warfarin, chlorpromazine, clindamycin and quinidine.

Capacity-limited binding insensitive drugs are those that have a low affinity for plasma proteins.

Examples include: Theophylline, chloramphenicol and paracetamol.

It is apparent that the opportunities for liver disease to influence drug elimination are greater and more complex than the opportunities afforded by renal disease. Not only is the kinetic behaviour of the particular drug of great importance, but the type of liver disease is also critical. In acute viral hepatitis the major change is in hepatocellular function. Drug metabolising ability usually remains intact and hepatic blood flow can actually increase. Mild to moderate cirrhosis tends to result in a decreased hepatic blood flow and portosystemic shunting, while severe cirrhosis usually shows reductions both in cellular function and blood flow.

Examples of what can happen to commonly used drugs are as follows: Pethidine and lignocaine both show flow-limited clearance. Not surprisingly, therefore, the clearance of both these drugs is unchanged in acute viral hepatitis, but reduced by about 50% in cirrhosis.

Phenytoin is cleared by a capacity-limited, binding-sensitive mechanism and here the effect on elimination depends on the balance between liver drug metabolising activity and protein binding. If there is reduced protein binding but little change in drug metabolising capacity, as in viral hepatitis, the total phenytoin concentration falls but the free drug concentration is unchanged. As in the case of renal failure, the therapeutic range must be set at a lower level. If, in addition, drug metabolising capacity is reduced free drug concentration actually rises leading to toxicity even at concentrations around the lower end of the usual therapeutic range.

Similar arguments apply to tolbutamide, diazepam and clindamycin.

Comment

Unlike the measurement of creatinine clearance in renal disease, there is no simple test that can predict the extent to which drug metabolism is decreased in liver disease. At best, a low serum albumin, raised bilirubin and prolonged prothrombin time give a rough guide.

The fact that a drug is metabolised by the liver does not necessarily mean that its kinetics are altered by liver disease, e.g. oxazepam disposition is normal both in hepatitis and cirrhosis. It is not possible, therefore, to extrapolate the findings from one drug to another. This is presumably because superficially similar metabolic pathways are mediated by different forms of cytochrome P450.

The documentation of modestly altered kinetics does not necessarily imply clinical importance. Even normal subjects show quite wide variations in kinetic indices and, in addition, kinetics should not be viewed in isolation from alterations in drug effect, which are usually much more difficult to assess. However, if a drug is known to be subject to substantial kinetic changes, then clinical significance is much more likely.

If it is clinically desirable to give a drug that is eliminated by liver metabolism to a patient with cirrhosis, it should be started in a low dose and drug levels or effect should be monitored very closely.

Altered pharmacodynamics

Deranged brain metabolism

The more severe forms of liver disease are accompanied by poorly understood derangements of brain metabolism, which ultimately result in the syndrome of hepatic encephalopathy. However, even before encephalopathy develops, the brain is extremely sensitive to the effects of centrally acting drugs.

This is independent of changes in drug kinetics. Coma can result from administering 'normal' doses of opiates or barbiturates to such patients.

Decreased clotting factors

Patients with liver disease also show increased sensitivity to oral anticoagulants. These drugs exert their effect by decreasing the vitamin K dependent synthesis of clotting factors II, VII, IX and X. When the production of these factors is already reduced by liver disease, a given dose of oral anticoagulant has a greater effect than in subjects with normal liver function.

Worsening of metabolic state

Drug-induced alkalosis

Excessive use of diuretics can precipitate encephalopathy. The mechanism involves hypokalaemic alkalosis, which results in conversion of NH_4^+ to NH_3, the unchanged ammonia crossing easily into the CNS to worsen or precipitate encephalopathy.

Fluid overload

Patients with advanced liver disease often have oedema and ascites secondary to hypoalbuminaemia and portal hypertension. This problem can be worsened by drugs that cause fluid retention, e.g. carbenoxolone, antacids that contain large amounts of sodium, and non steroidal anti-inflammatory agents. (This last group of drugs should be avoided anyway because of the increased risk of gastrointestinal bleeding.)

TABLE 2.2   Drugs that can cause liver damage

HEPATITIS
    Halothane (repeated exposure)
    Isoniazid
    Methyldopa
    Phenelzine

CHOLESTASIS with a mild hepatic component
    Phenothiazines
    Tricyclic antidepressants
    Nonsteroidal anti-inflammatory drugs (especially phenylbutazone)
    Rifampicin, ethambutol, pyrazinamide
    Sulphonylureas
    Sulphonamides, ampicillin, nitrofurantoin;
       erythromycin estolate
    Oral contraceptive (stasis without hepatitis)

CIRRHOSIS
    Methotrexate

Hepatotoxic drugs (Table 2.2)

Where an acceptable alternative exists, it is wise to avoid drugs that can cause liver damage, e.g. oral contraceptives, rifampicin, and repeated exposure to halothane anaesthesia.

2.4   INFLUENCE OF CONGESTIVE HEART FAILURE

Congestive heart failure can influence drug kinetics in the following ways:

(1) Decreased rate or extent of gastrointestinal absorption, e.g. procainamide and hydrochlorthiazide.

(2) Decreased volume of distribution, e.g. lignocaine and procainamide.

(3) Decreased elimination, e.g. lignocaine, theophylline.

Decreased gastrointestinal absorption

The main factors involved are:

(1) mucosal oedema,

(2) reduced epithelial blood supply,

(3) splanchnic vasoconstriction.

Procainamide bioavailability can be reduced by up to 50% and figures of 30–40% have been reported for the diuretics hydrochlorthiazide and metolazone.

Frusemide absorption is delayed but bioavailability is not reduced.

Decreased volume of distribution

This is thought to result from decreased tissue perfusion. It is clearly documented for two drugs: lignocaine (reduced by about 50% in severe failure), and procainamide (reduced by about 25%). Therefore, for any given dose, correspondingly higher blood concentrations are achieved. The corollary and practical importance of this is that initial loading doses should be correspondingly reduced.

Decreased elimination

The main factors involved are, for the liver:
  (1) Decreased perfusion,
  (2) Decreased oxidising capacity because of hypoxia,
  (3) Decreased metabolizing capacity because of congestion;

and for the kidney:
  (1) Decreased glomerular filtration rate,
  (2) increased tubular reabsorption.

The clearance of lignocaine is dependent on liver blood flow and in heart failure can be reduced by up to 50%. For theophylline the metabolic capacity of the liver is important and again clearance is reduced in heart failure. Procainamide is cleared mainly unchanged by renal excretion with about 20% being converted to the active metabolite N-acetylprocainamide (NAPA) which is subsequently excreted by the kidney. In heart failure both procainamide and NAPA show reduced elimination.

These drugs all have concentration related toxicity. Therefore:
  (1) The rate of administration must be reduced in heart failure,
  (2) Drug concentration monitoring is highly desirable.

2.5   INFLUENCE OF THYROID DISEASE

Thyroid disease alters a patient's response to digoxin. Hyperthyroid patients are relatively resistant to the drug while hypothyroid patients are extremely sensitive to it. The reasons are in part kinetic and in part dynamic. The clearance of digoxin is roughly proportional to thyroid function so for any given dose, lower concentrations are achieved in hyperthyroid patients and higher concentrations are achieved in hypothyroid patients compared to normals. In addition, hypothyroidism increases the sensitivity of cardiac tissue to digoxin but the mechanism is not understood.

Lithium can cause hypothyroidism apparently by inhibiting release of thyroid hormone from the gland. It is important to recognise this complication in order to avoid mistaking hypothyroidism for a relapse in the depressive illness. Thyroxine can be prescribed concurrently with lithium.

CHAPTER 3

Drugs at the extremes of age

Most information in clinical pharmacology has been derived from experiments and observations in young or middle-aged patients or healthy volunteers. However, most drug use is concentrated in children and in those over the age of 65 years. In Scotland, for example, approximately 20% of prescriptions are issued for those aged less than 16 years and 40% for those over 65 years. Very little information is available about drug absorption, effect and elimination at these extremes of age.

3.1   USE OF DRUGS IN NEONATES

Drug distribution

Compared to the adult a much higher percentage of neonatal body mass is water: 75% is water in the full-term neonate, while 85% is the figure in premature babies. In a premature infant only 1% of body weight is accounted for by fat, while in the full-term neonate the figure is 15%.

Membrane permeability is generally greater in the neonate compared to the adult, and this is particularly true of the blood–brain barrier.

Protein binding is considerably less in the neonate compared to the adult. Possible reasons for this include the presence of competing endogenous substances (bilirubin, free fatty acids, steroids) differences in pH and differences in the molecular species of binding proteins. A decrease in protein binding and increased volume of distribution have been demonstrated in the neonate for salicylates, benzylpenicillin, ampicillin and digoxin.

Drug metabolism

Liver drug metabolising activity is reduced in the neonate, but it is difficult to generalise as different pathways develop at different rates. Hydroxylation and glucuronidation are very slow to develop while sulphate conjugation is much faster. Many commonly used drugs have been shown to have substantially prolonged half-lives in the neonate: diazepam, phenobarbitone, nortriptyline, tolbutamide, theophylline and chloramphenicol. The decreased metabolism of chloramphenicol can cause an adverse reaction characterised by cardiovascular collapse, coma and cyanosis.

Drug excretion

Glomerular filtration at birth is approximately 30–40% that of the adult when corrected for body surface area, while at the fifth day of life glomerular filtration rate has increased to about 50% of adult values. This decreased renal function has the predictable effect of decreasing the clearance of drugs that undergo renal elimination. Benzylpenicillin is cleared from premature infants at around 30% of the rate seen in adults when adjusted for body weight. The same observations have been made with other penicillins and the aminoglycosides.

Drug effect

One method of assessing drug effect is to compare the LD_{50} in neonatal and mature animals. Using this technique various central nervous system depressants such as barbiturates, chlorpromazine and the opiates have been shown to have substantially greater effect on a mg/kg dose basis in neonatal compared to mature animals. On the other hand, some clinically important drugs are less potent in the neonate: for example, digoxin and phenytoin. The increased volume of distribution of digoxin cannot by itself explain the greater dose per kg needed in the neonate since studies on isolated cardiac tissue shown that there is intrinsic decrease in sensitivity to digoxin in the neonatal period. Therefore, these drugs are given on a greater mg/kg dose regimen than is true in the adult.

Comment

These differences in distribution, elimination and effect between neonates and adults, between premature and full-term neonates, and between drugs in babies of the same maturity mean that no hard and fast rules can be applied to drug dosing. In general, effective and safe doses have been arrived at by experience, and guidance is found in standard textbooks of paediatrics.

3.2 USE OF DRUGS IN CHILDREN

Drug metabolism

Several drugs that are cleared by liver metabolism undergo more rapid elimination in late infancy and early childhood compared to the adult.

Examples include: phenytoin, theophylline, carbamazepine and phenobarbitone.

Drug excretion

Glomerular filtration reaches adult rates by about 5 months of age while tubular secretion and reabsorption achieve adult levels by about 7 months. Digoxin appears to have a greater clearance in children than adults: the effective daily dose in childhood is around 10–15 μg/kg compared with approximately 3.5 μg/kg in adults.

Therapeutic drug concentration monitoring

The indication for drug concentration monitoring should be the same as in adults. However, the results must be interpreted in the light of considerable ignorance about concentration–effect relationships in children.

Drug doses

There is no entirely satisfactory method of calculating drug dose in children because of differences in elimination and possibly also drug effect compared to adults. It is certainly not satisfactory simply to scale down adult doses, since children generally need more on a mg/kg basis. Working from a knowledge of surface area tends to be more reliable, but this requires estimation from nomograms after obtaining height and weight:

$$\text{dose} = \frac{\text{surface area } (m^2)}{1.8} \times \text{adult dose}$$

However, this should still be regarded as an approximation.

Comment

For most commonly used drugs detailed guidelines are available in textbooks and practical guides to paediatrics. *If you are prescribing for a child, check the dose schedule first.*

3.3 USE OF DRUGS IN THE ELDERLY

The transition from middle to old age is accompanied by substantial changes both in body composition and body function with the result that there are alterations both in drug disposition and effect. In addition the frequency and severity of adverse drug reactions increases with age as does the problem of noncompliance with drug therapy.

Drug absorption

Age related changes in upper gastrointestinal function (achlorhydria, changes in motility or diminished blood flow) may modify absorption. However, these effects have not yet been shown to have clinical significance.

Drug distribution

In old age there is a considerable increase in the ratio of adipose to lean tissue, while total body weight tends to decrease. In addition there is a decrease in serum albumin concentration. These changes would be expected to result in an increased volume of distribution of many drugs and the evidence supports this: diazepam, lignocaine, chlormethiazole and prazosin have all been shown to have an increased volume of distribution in the elderly.

Drug metabolism

In experimental animals increasing age is associated with a reduction in liver microsomal drug metabolising activity. In man, total liver weight and the number of functioning liver cells has been shown to decrease with increasing age. One might expect that increasing age would be associated with decreasing clearance of those drugs which undergo metabolism but, as in the neonate, different metabolic pathways are influenced to a different extent by age. Thus the clearance of diazepam, lignocaine, nitrazepam, nortriptyline, paracetamol and warfarin is not affected by age. On the other hand, chlormethiazole undergoes decreased clearance in the elderly.

Renal elimination of drugs

Renal function decreases with age. Glomerular filtration rate, tubular secretion, reabsorptive capacity and renal blood flow all decrease linearly from the age of 30. Several drugs that are eliminated by the kidney have prolonged half-lives in the elderly: digoxin, benzylpenicillin, gentamicin. As a rule, these drugs must be prescribed in lower doses in older people.

Drug effect in the elderly

There is strong evidence that the responsiveness of beta adrenoceptors decreases in the elderly, both to agonists and antagonists. There is less evidence concerning the sensitivity of elderly subjects to benzodiazepines. However, it is likely that elderly subjects are more sensitive to these drugs independent of any changes in absorption or distribution. Elderly people are more sensitive to the anticoagulant effects of warfarin, but the mechanism of this has not been defined. Related to the question of drug sensitivity is the physiological response to drug action. In the case of drugs that lower blood pressure, for example, the reflex response to a given fall in pressure substantially decreases with age with the result that drug effect can be greatly enhanced. Similarly, the effect of various diuretics is greater in the elderly.

Prescribing in the elderly

Adverse drug reactions occur more frequently in the elderly. Between the ages of 20 and 29 years, 3% of patients experience adverse drug reactions: this percentage rises to 21% for the age range 70–79. The reasons for this include:

(1) The number of drugs prescribed increases with age, increasing not only the chance of an adverse drug reaction but also of an adverse drug interaction.

(2) Doses used are sometimes too high in relation to reduced elimination, e.g. digoxin.

(3) Doses used are sometimes too high in relation to decreased physiological responses, e.g. hypotensive drugs.

Compliance with drug therapy can be a problem in the elderly particularly if the drug regimen is complex and if the patient does not understand why the drug is being prescribed. Failing eye sight and decreased power in the hands can be very simple but important reasons why the patient is not taking the drugs prescribed.

Therapeutic drug monitoring

As for children, it may not be appropriate to extrapolate concentration–effect relationships from middle-aged patients to the elderly. Caution is advisable when interpreting concentration values.

Comment

When prescribing for an elderly person start with a low dose and increase slowly if necessary. Keep treatment as simple as possible employing the minimum number of different drugs. Make sure the patient or a responsible person clearly understands the treatment schedule. Avoid childproof containers for those who are unable to open them. Remember that if an elderly person is unwell for no obvious reason, drugs may be the cause and a dramatic improvement may occur if all drugs are withdrawn.

CHAPTER 4

Drugs in pregnant and breast-feeding women

4.1 Effect of drugs on the fetus

4.2 Effect of pregnancy on drug absorption, distribution and elimination

4.3 Drug treatment of common medical problems during pregnancy

4.4 Breast feeding

Women in the United Kingdom each take an average of four drugs during pregnancy, excluding iron, and drugs used during delivery. Once in the maternal circulation, drugs are separated from the fetus by a lipid placental membrane which any given drug crosses to a greater or lesser extent depending on the physicochemical properties of the molecule.

Drugs in pregnancy can be viewed from two standpoints:
(1) Effect of drugs on the fetus,
(2) Effect of pregnancy on the drug.

4.1 EFFECT OF DRUGS ON THE FETUS

Drugs can influence fetal development at three separate stages:
(1) Fertilisation and implantation period—conception to about 17 days gestation
(2) Organogenesis—18–55 days
(3) Growth and development—56 days onward.

The possible consequences of drug exposure are quite different at each stage.

Fertilisation and implantation period

Interference by a drug with either of these processes clearly leads to failure of the pregnancy at a very early and probably subclinical stage. Therefore, very little is known about drugs that influence this process in the human.

Organogenesis

It is during this period that the developing embryo shows great sensitivity to the teratogenic effects of drugs. A teratogen is any substance (virus, environmental toxin, or drug) that produces deformity. Before discussing the teratogenic properties of certain drugs, the following points must be appreciated.

(1) Teratogenesis in the human is very difficult to predict from animal studies because of considerable species variation. Thalidomide, the most notorious drug teratogen of recent times, showed no teratogenicity in mice and rats.

(2) Serious congenital deformities are present in 1–2% of all babies. Therefore, a drug is only readily identified as teratogenic if its effects are frequent, unusual and/or serious. A low-grade teratogen that infrequently causes minor deformities is likely to pass unnoticed.

TABLE 4.1   Drugs that are contraindicated in pregnancy because of teratogenesis

Drug	Deformity
Androgens	Virilisation, limb reduction, oesophageal anomalies, cardiac defects.
Diethylstilboestrol	Adenocarcinoma of vagina in teenage years
Tetracyclines	Inhibition of bone growth; discolouration of teeth
Methotrexate	Multiple defects
Oral anticoagulants	Bone abnormalities, saddle nose, optic atrophy, mental retardation
Oral hypoglycaemics	Multiple anomalies

Table 4.1 lists drugs that are contraindicated in pregnancy because they are definitely teratogenic. In many other instances a drug has been implicated in teratogenesis, but confirmatory evidence has usually been lacking.

Comment

The greatest risk of teratogenesis occurs at a time when a woman might not even be aware that she is pregnant. Only a few drugs are known definitely to be teratogenic, but many more could be under certain circumstances. When prescribing for a woman of childbearing age remember that she might be pregnant and ask yourself if the benefits of drug use outweigh the risks, however, small, of teratogenesis.

Growth and development

During this stage major body structures have been formed, and it is their subsequent development and function that can be affected:

(1) Antithyroid drugs (Chapter 20.2) cross the placenta and can cause fetal and neonatal hypothyroidism.

(2) Prostaglandin synthetase inhibitors, e.g. indomethacin; aspirin in high dose, can cause premature closure of the ductus arteriosus with substantial neonatal mortality.

(3) Drugs with a CNS depressant action, such as opiates and benzodiazepines, are often given at the very end of pregnancy or during labour. If excessive doses are used neonatal hypotension, respiratory depression and hypothermia can occur.

(4) Drugs with dependence potential, e.g. opiates, and dextropropoxyphene, which are taken regularly during pregnancy can result in withdrawal symptoms in the neonate.

4.2 EFFECT OF PREGNANCY ON DRUG ABSORPTION, DISTRIBUTION AND ELIMINATION

The substantial physiological changes that occur in pregnancy can influence drug disposition while pathological conditions in pregnancy can accentuate these changes.

Absorption

There is a decrease in gastrointestinal motility during the later part of pregnancy, and this can either increase the absorption of poorly soluble drugs such as digoxin or decrease the absorption of drugs that undergo metabolism in the gut wall, such as chlorpromazine.

Drug distribution

Maternal plasma volume and extracellular fluid volume increases by about 50% by the last trimester, and this should decrease the steady state concentration of drugs with a small volume of distribution. Considerable changes in protein concentration occur during the last trimester with serum albumin falling by about 20% while alpha$_1$ acid glycoprotein increases in concentration by about 40% in normal pregnancies. These changes are accentuated in pre-eclampsia with albumin concentration falling by about 34% and glycoprotein rising by as much as 100%. This means that the free fraction of acidic drugs can substantially increase while that of basic drugs can be greatly decreased in the last trimester. Diazepam, phenytoin and sodium valproate have been shown to have significantly elevated free fractions in the last trimester.

Drug elimination

Effective renal plasma flow has doubled by the end of pregnancy and this would be expected to increase the elimination of polar drugs which undergo renal elimination. The hepatic microsomal mixed function oxidase system undergoes induction in pregnancy, probably as the result of high circulating levels of progesterone. This leads to an increased clearance of drugs that undergo metabolism by this pathway, and there is evidence that the steady state concentrations of the anticonvulsants sodium valproate, phenytoin, carbamazepine and phenobarbitone are decreased to a clinically significant extent in the last trimester. Therefore, higher doses are required as the pregnancy progresses, with careful monitoring of drug concentrations. An unknown factor in drug clearance during pregnancy is the contribution made by the placenta. Most major drug metabolising systems have been identified in the placenta but their contribution has yet to be defined.

4.3 DRUG TREATMENT OF COMMON MEDICAL PROBLEMS DURING PREGNANCY

Infection

Urinary tract infections are common during pregnancy. Penicillins are the preferred treatment (subject to appropriate sensitivity testing), since these drugs have never been implicated in teratogenesis. Tetracyclines are contraindicated (Table 4.1). Co-trimoxazole should be avoided. In early pregnancy the trimethoprim component can possibly cause cleft palate, while at the end of pregnancy the sulphonamide component can cross the placenta and displace bilirubin from protein binding sites in the neonate.

Severe infections in pregnancy are fortunately rare. Aminoglycosides cause fetal eighth nerve damage, and the benefits of their use must be seen in this context. At present there is no evidence to suggest fetal damage from cephalosporins, metronidazole or chloramphenicol. However, chloramphenicol can cause cardiovascular collapse in neonates and should not be used at the end of pregnancy.

In the case of tuberculosis, both isoniazid and ethambutol have been used extensively during pregnancy, including the first trimester, with no fetal defects. The incidence of fetal deformity following rifampicin is three times greater than with isoniazid or ethambutol, but still within the normal range. Streptomycin definitely causes auditory deficit and should not be used.

Diabetes mellitus

Diabetic pregnancies are associated with a twofold increase in perinatal mortality. Liveborn neonates are prone to respiratory distress syndrome, hypoglycaemia, hypocalcaemia and jaundice.

The aim of therapy is *obsessionally* to maintain pre-prandial blood glucose concentrations between 3 and 6 mmol/l (55–110 mg/100 ml). The adequacy of therapy in the short term is monitored by daily pre-prandial glucose estimation either in hospital or at home using capillary blood on glucose oxidase impregnated sticks.

Gestational diabetes, i.e. the development of mild glucose intolerance during pregnancy, can sometimes be managed adequately by carbohydrate restriction. If this fails, insulin is used.

Insulin is usually given as twice daily injections of a highly purified preparation containing a mixture of short and intermediate acting types (p. 291). Insulin-dependent diabetics who are on different regimens should be changed when they become pregnant or, preferably, before conception. Oral hypoglycaemics are teratogenic and have no place in managing diabetic pregnancies. Insulin requirements often increase from around the fifteenth to thirtieth week of pregnancy, remain constant until delivery and then fall rapidly to pre-pregnancy levels. Therefore, daily monitoring of blood glucose is mandatory to maintain normoglycaemia.

Asthma

Poorly controlled asthma is associated with increased perinatal mortality. Maternal hypoxia and respiratory alkalosis are the major determinants of fetal distress in asthmatic pregnancies.

Theophylline, salbutamol by metered aerosol, and steroids have good safety records at all stages of pregnancy. There has been little experience with newer bronchodilators.

Pregnancy should not alter the general approach to asthma as described in Chapter 10.1. It is important to control bronchospasm and avoid prolonged abnormalities of blood gases or acid–base balance.

Epilepsy

The main issues are possible *teratogenicity* associated with anticonvulsants and the need for *therapeutic drug level monitoring* to control fits.

Sodium valproate and carbamazepine both appear to be free of teratogenic effects in humans and whenever possible should be used to treat female epileptics of childbearing age. Phenytoin appears to be teratogenic and may cause craniofacial and distal limb abnormalities. However, the teratogenicity of phenytoin has not been conclusively demonstrated, and there is no widely accepted policy for dealing with a woman who wishes to become pregnant and is well controlled on phenytoin. The majority view at present is that phenytoin should be continued since the risk to the fetus of uncontrolled epilepsy almost certainly equals those of phenytoin. Phenobarbitone also may be teratogenic.

The pharmacokinetic changes associated with pregnancy are clinically important in the treatment of epilepsy. Anticonvulsant concentrations tend to fall during pregnancy (see above) and, although partially offset by a decrease in protein binding, this change in drug level can be accompanied by increased seizure frequency. Therefore, concentration monitoring is required at monthly intervals during pregnancy. The aim should be to maintain concentrations at the lower end of the therapeutic range, with doses being increased as necessary to achieve this. Postpartum there is a return to normal kinetics over 5–10 days and monitoring is again required to aid dosage adjustment.

Hypertension

Maternal high blood pressure is a leading cause of fetal loss, particularly when it is severe or accompanied by proteinuria. In addition, hypertension is the leading (though rare) cause of maternal death in the U.K.

Bed rest and sedation have traditionally been used but neither is of proven value.

Among antihypertensive drugs, methyldopa has been most widely used. It significantly lowers blood pressure and reduces midtrimester abortions in patients with essential hypertension, but has not been shown to influence fetal outcome in hypertension developing later in pregnancy. Methyldopa is not teratogenic.

Beta-blockers successfully lower blood pressure in pregnancy, but have not been shown conclusively to improve fetal outcome. They are not teratogenic.

Hydralazine is often used to complement one of the above drugs and similarly causes no damage to the fetus but is of uncertain value in improving fetal outcome.

Diuretics are contraindicated in the management of hypertension during pregnancy because such patients are already volume depleted and diuresis can further impair perfusion of the fetoplacental unit.

Hyperthyroidism

Carbimazole crosses the placenta and appears in breast milk. The concentrations achieved in the fetus or neonate are sufficient to suppress thyroid function. Various approaches have been advocated:

(1) the use of the lowest dose of carbimazole that controls the hyperthyroidism and reducing this towards term,

(2) the administration of a beta blocker alone to provide symptomatic relief until other treatment can be instituted after delivery,

(3) or partial thyroidectomy if the condition is diagnosed in the first trimester.

4.4 BREAST FEEDING

Breast feeding has become popular again in Western countries. It deepens the emotional relationship between mother and baby, confers some protection against infections in early life and lowers the incidence of the sudden infant death syndrome. The factors that determine the transfer of drugs into breast milk are the same as those influencing drug distribution in general (Chapter 1.3).

Most drugs enter breast milk to a greater or lesser extent but, because the concentration has been greatly reduced by distribution throughout the mother's body, the amount of drug actually received by the breast-fed baby is usually clinically insignificant.

Drugs that can safely be given to breast-feeding mothers include:
Penicillins, cephalosporins.
Theophylline, salbutamol by inhaler, prednisolone.
Valproate, carbamazepine, phenytoin;
Beta blockers, methyldopa, hydralazine.
Warfarin, heparin.
Haloperidol, chlorpromazine.
Tricyclic antidepressants.
Oral contraceptives (low oestrogen dose).

Certain drugs achieve sufficient concentration in breast milk, and they are sufficiently potent that their use in breast feeding mothers should be avoided:
Sulphonamides, chloramphenicol, isoniazid; tetracyclines.
Narcotic analgesics.
Benzodiazepines.
Lithium.
Antithyroid drugs, radioactive iodine.

Comment

If a lactating woman requires drug therapy, it is nearly always safe to proceed both with breast feeding and drug administration. Only infrequently is a drug other than those listed above considered. However, if the proposed treatment is with an agent which is not often used, obtain further information before proceeding.

CHAPTER 5

Clinical pharmacokinetics: therapeutic drug monitoring

5.1   Justification for therapeutic drug monitoring

5.2   Variability in drug disposition

5.3   Interpretation of plasma levels

Optimum treatment with many drugs depends on achieving a
plasma concentration that lies between specific limits set by a
minimum effective concentration (MEC) and a maximum safe
concentration (MSC). There may be some dispute about the most
appropriate values for these limits, but concentrations lying above
the MSC are usually associated with toxicity while those lying
below the MEC are generally ineffective. It is the aim of
therapeutic drug monitoring to ensure that drug concentrations lie
between these limits, i.e. within the *therapeutic range*.

As patients vary widely in the ways in which they absorb,
distribute, metabolise and eliminate many drugs, dosage in these
circumstances merits individual consideration. This can be assisted
by the measurement of drug levels in the blood because a
'standard' or 'average' dose results in toxic effects in some patients
and less than ideal treatment in others.

5.1   JUSTIFICATION FOR THERAPEUTIC DRUG MONITORING

In some instances, the most appropriate dose of a drug for an
individual can be selected by titrating it against a readily

38

measurable response. This approach, without the need of plasma concentration measurements, is adopted with the following classes of drugs:

Anticoagulants,
Antihypertensives,
Analgesics,
Hypoglycaemics,
Diuretics.

In each case, a clearly identifiable target response can be measured and the achievement of this outweighs more indirect assessments based on plasma concentrations. In other cases, either because the target response is more difficult to quantify, or because the therapeutic range, which may be quite narrow, has been clearly defined, measurement of plasma concentrations can be extremely valuable. This approach is justified with the following drugs:

Drugs to control cardiac arrhythmias (Chapter 6.1)

Digoxin,
Disopyramide,
Lignocaine,
Procainamide,
N-acetyl procainamide,
Mexiletine,
Quinidine.

Anticonvulsants (Chapter 19.1)

Phenytoin,
Carbamazepine,
Phenobarbitone,
Primidone,
Sodium valproate.

Antibiotics (Chapter 9.2)

Gentamicin,
Tobramycin,
Amikacin.

Miscellaneous

Theophylline (Chapter 10.1),
Methotrexate (Chapter 12.1),
Lithium (Chapter 18.5).

The justification depends on the fact that there are a number of clear reasons why concentrations achieved with these drugs may be unpredictable, the most important ones being:

(1) Wide interindividual variability in drug disposition including nonlinear pharmacokinetics.

(2) The presence of gastrointestinal, cardiac, hepatic or renal disease (Chapter 2).

(3) Poor patient compliance (Chapter 26).

(4) Suspected drug interactions.

5.2   VARIABILITY IN DRUG DISPOSITION

Drug disposition is a term used to describe the movement of a drug throughout the body. The various processes involved, absorption, distribution, metabolism and excretion, differ from individual to individual. These *pharmacokinetic* differences must be accounted for when tailoring doses to achieve specific target concentrations. The most important determinants of this variability are:

(1) Volume of distribution,

(2) Clearance.

Volume of distribution

As a drug enters the systemic circulation it distributes widely throughout the blood and extravascular fluids to binding sites, target organs and organs of elimination. Binding sites include those within the circulation, the plasma proteins, and those dispersed throughout the tissues, of both a specific and a non-specific nature. Movement of drug between the blood and all other sites proceeds until an equilibrium is established when the concentration of drug in plasma water equals that of the drug in tissue fluids.

Drug distribution is interpreted mathematically as the volume of fluid into which the drug *apparently* distributes. This so called *apparent volume of distribution* (V_d) need not refer to any real, physiological volume, but it is merely *the volume that would accommodate all drug in the body if its concentration throughout the body was the same as that in the plasma.* Therefore, at equilibrium it is easy to see that this volume is determined by the *amount* of drug in the body and the *associated plasma concentration*:

$$V_d = \frac{\text{Amount of drug in body}}{\text{plasma concentration}}$$

This assumes that, as far as the drug is concerned, the body acts as a single homogeneous compartment. Bearing this assumption in mind, V_d can be determined by measuring a number of plasma concentrations after a single intravenous injection of a drug, and calculating the theoretical concentration that occurred at the moment of injection, or Cp_o. Cp_o is obtained by extrapolating the semi-logarithmic plot of concentration against time to the y axis as shown in Fig. 5.1. Then:

$$V_d = \frac{\text{Intravenous dose}}{Cp_o}$$

Conversely, V_d can be used to calculate the amount of drug in the body when the plasma concentration is known or to predict the concentration in the plasma following a known dose.

The V_d for a particular drug within a particular individual is determined largely by:
 (1) The degree of lipid solubility of the drug,
 (2) The degree of binding to plasma and tissue proteins.
A small apparent V_d is favoured by:
 (1) Low lipid solubility,
 (2) A high degree of plasma protein binding,
 (3) A low level of tissue binding.
A high apparent V_d is favoured by:
 (1) Increased lipid solubility,
 (2) Reduced plasma protein binding,
 (3) Increased tissue binding.
Some of the reasons why V_d is important have been presented in Chapter 1.3. Additionally it is used to:
 (1) Calculate the size of a *loading dose*,
 (2) Estimate the fluctuations in plasma levels (peaks and troughs) which occur with repetitive dosing. This also requires a knowledge of clearance.

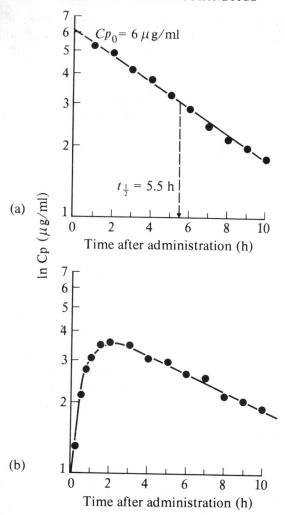

FIG. 5.1 Examples of plasma concentration–time profiles after (a) intravenous and (b) oral administration.

Calculation of loading dose

A loading dose may sometimes be appropriate at the outset of treatment if an immediate response is required and the concentration–response relationship has been clearly defined. It is possible, for example, to start digoxin therapy with a loading dose so that *therapeutic levels* can be achieved within hours instead of 3–4 days. An intravenous loading dose is calculated as follows:

$$\text{Loading dose} = V_d \times \text{desired plasma concentration}$$

This simply recognises that the dose given is distributed throughout the volume of distribution and to achieve the desired concentration *in the plasma* (whose volume may be considerably less than the V_d), the desired concentration must be multiplied by the total volume of distribution.

Peak and trough levels

It may be important to estimate the plasma concentration during repetitive drug administration principally in terms of the *peak* (maximum) and *trough* (minimum) levels achieved. This is determined by the size of the dose, the volume of distribution, and clearance. Ideally, dose regimens should be designed to maintain concentrations within the therapeutic range so that peak levels do not exceed the MSC and trough levels do not fall below the MEC.

The differences in volumes of distribution between individuals can usually be accounted for by differences in one or other easily identifiable physiological variables such as actual body weight or lean body mass. Therefore, it is relatively easy to make a good estimate of the volume of distribution in an individual patient.

Clearance

Most drug regimens call for repetitive administration over varying periods of time, and if consistent and safe levels in the blood and the body are to be achieved, a balance must be struck between the amount prescribed (input) and the amount eliminated (output). The input–output balance is controlled by the clinician who must decide on the most appropriate dosage regimen that offsets the elimination of the drug in an individual patient.

A useful concept which describes this balance and which embraces drug loss from the body is *clearance*. When the rate of administration (R_{in}) equals the rate of elimination (R_{out}), *steady state* has been achieved. R_{in} can be calculated as follows:

$$R_{in} = \frac{F \cdot \text{Dose}}{\tau}$$

F, which has a value between 0 and 1, is an estimate of the proportion of drug actually absorbed (its bioavailability), and τ is the time over which the drug is administered, i.e. the dosage interval. Clearance (Cl) can be thought of as a proportionality factor which relates average steady-state plasma levels $(\overline{Cp_{ss}})$ to the rate of drug administration, thus

$$R_{in} = Cl \cdot \overline{Cp}_{ss}$$

then

$$\frac{F \cdot \text{Dose}}{\tau} = Cl \cdot \overline{Cp}_{ss}$$

If $\overline{Cp_{ss}}$ is known, clearance can be calculated by rearranging this equation:

$$Cl = \frac{F \cdot \text{Dose}}{\overline{Cp}_{ss} \cdot \tau}$$

It is important to note that from a practical point of view, $\overline{Cp_{ss}}$ can be estimated as the concentration which is approximately midway between the maximum and minimum concentrations at steady state.

Clearance is expressed in units of volume per time. This emphasises that it does not portray the *amount* of drug being eliminated but the *theoretical volume of blood or plasma from which drug is completely removed in a given period of time*. Its utility lies in the fact that if both the clearance and the desired steady-state concentration are known, then it is easy to calculate the appropriate dose, again by rearranging the above equation:

$$\text{Dose} = \frac{Cl \cdot \overline{Cp}_{ss} \cdot \tau}{F}$$

With an intravenous infusion, F is 1.0 and the equation reduces to:

$$\text{Dose} = Cl \cdot \overline{Cp}_{ss} \cdot \tau$$

In clinical practice, these equations have one very important implication: *dose and steady-state concentration are directly proportional*. Doubling the dose should lead to a twofold increase in $\overline{Cp_{ss}}$ and halving the dose leads to half the original $\overline{Cp_{ss}}$. This simple relationship holds for most drugs and in pharmacokinetic terms, is known as a *first-order*, or *linear process*. This has already been referred to in relation to drug metabolism in Chapter 1.4. It is

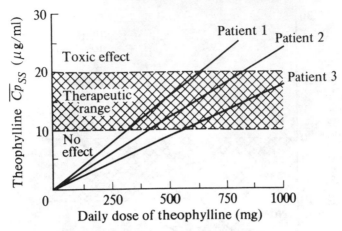

F IG . 5.2   Diagrammatic illustration of different dose–concentration relationships where drug clearance is a first-order process.

illustrated in Fig. 5.2, where the bronchodilator drug theophylline is used as an example.

There are one or two notable exceptions, when the dose–$\overline{Cp}_{ss}$ relationship is *not* linear, and it is then referred to as a *zero-order process*. An increase in $\overline{Cp}_{ss}$ occurs out of all proportion to an increase in dose. This is illustrated in Fig. 5.3 and is exemplified by the anticonvulsant phenytoin. A proportionality between dose and steady-state concentration may exist up to a certain point, which may vary from individual to individual, but beyond this point, concentrations rise very steeply meaning that very small increments in dose produce excessively large, potentially toxic, increases in plasma concentration. This is because the hepatic enzyme system which metabolises phenytoin becomes saturated at a certain substrate level, often at a concentration within the therapeutic range. At this point, when the linear relationship breaks down, the enzymes no longer metabolise the drug at a rate proportional to the substrate concentration, but at a constant rate. This is reflected by the associated steep rise in plasma concentrations.

Utility of clearance estimates

The majority of drugs obey first-order kinetics and it may be very useful to obtain an estimate of clearance in individual patients. Measurement of a steady-state drug level can be used to calculate

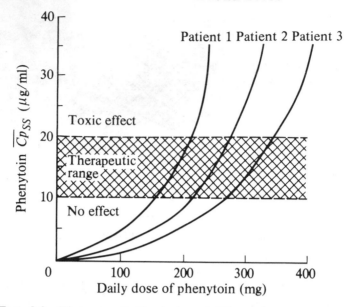

FIG. 5.3 Diagrammatic illustration of different dose–concentration relationships where drug clearance is predominantly a zero-order process.

clearance as is shown above, and this can then be used to calculate a dose that achieves a desired concentration. This approach has highlighted the differences in clearance that exist both between individuals and in the *same* individual at different points in time.

Clearance of the bronchodilator theophylline for example, can be influenced by:

Age,
Weight,
Diet,
Alcohol consumption,
Smoking,
Other drugs,
Diseases such as:
    Cardiac failure,
    Hepatic cirrhosis,
    Pulmonary oedema.

Clearance, therefore, in any individual, results from the balance between various factors and is difficult to determine in the absence of plasma concentration measurements. Good estimates, however, can be made if significant relationships have been established between drug clearance and the many patient factors listed above. For drugs primarily excreted by the kidney, e.g. digoxin and gentamicin, the creatinine clearance is the most important determinant of drug clearance. Thus digoxin clearance, in a 70 kg patient without cardiac failure, can be estimated from the equation:

$$\text{Digoxin clearance (ml/min)} = 1.02 \left(\frac{\text{Creatinine clearance}}{} \right) + 57 \ \text{ml/min}$$

If the patient has cardiac failure, the equation is modified thus:

$$\text{Digoxin clearance (ml/min)} = 0.88 \left(\frac{\text{Creatinine clearance}}{} \right) + 23 \ \text{ml/min}$$

Drug elimination and half-life

Just as the input–output balance has been described in terms of clearance, the output side of the equation can be quantified in a way that provides further useful information for the clinician. The linear relationship between dose and steady-state concentration is based on the fact that the rate of elimination of most drugs *is proportional to the drug concentration*. Thus the amount of drug eliminated per unit of time varies proportionately with drug concentration, but the fraction of the total amount of drug present in the body which is removed at any time remains constant and independent of the dose. Mathematically, this first-order elimination process implies that the amount or concentration of drug in the blood or body diminishes logarithmically with time (Fig. 5.1). The equation which describes this process is:

$$Cp(t) = Cp_o \, e^{-k_e t}$$

where $Cp(t)$ is the concentration at any time (t), Cp_o is the (theoretical) concentration at zero time (i.e. at the instant of injection), k_e is the *elimination rate constant*, and $e^{-k_e t}$ is the fraction of drug remaining at time t.

A plot of the natural logarithm of concentration against time yields a straight line (Fig. 5.1). The important point to note is that if the body can be conceived of as a single compartment, then after an intravenous injection the mathematical function that best fits the observed decline in plasma concentration is a single exponential with an equation of the form shown above. Input by another route, such as the gut, complicates matters because absorption takes an appreciable time and manifests itself in the shape of the concentration–time curve. Clearly, an increase in concentration during the absorption phase leads to a peak and then a decline, the shape of this curve being determined by the rates of absorption and elimination (Fig. 5.1b).

From the measurement of plasma levels it is possible to calculate the two unknown values, Cp_o and k_e, the *pharmacokinetic parameters*.

Cp_o has been defined above; k_e, the elimination rate constant, is the slope of the line in Fig. 5.1, and it is the fraction of the total amount of drug in the body which is removed per unit of time. It is, in turn, a function of clearance and volume of distribution, thus

$$k_e = \frac{Cl}{V_d}$$

Therefore k_e also expresses the fraction of the volume of distribution which is cleared of drug per unit of time. But as this is not particularly meaningful to the clinician, k_e can be more usefully expressed in terms of the *half-life* of a drug. *The half-life ($t\frac{1}{2}$) is the time required for the plasma concentration to fall to one-half of its original value* and is derived either graphically (see Fig. 5.1) or from the relationship:

$$t_{\frac{1}{2}} = \frac{\ln 2}{k_e}$$

where ln 2 is the natural logarithm of 2, or 0.693.

If the half-life of a drug is known—whether the figure represents an average value for the group of patients concerned or better still, an estimate of the value for an individual patient—it can be used to make predictions about treatment with that drug. It is useful to know at what time steady state is reached after starting a regular treatment schedule or after any change in dose. As a rule, steady state is attained after four-to-five half-lives. Further, when toxic drug levels have been inadvertently produced, it is very useful to estimate how long it takes for such levels to reach the therapeutic range; or how long it takes for all the drug to be eliminated once the drug has been stopped. Usually, elimination is effectively complete after four-to-five half-lives. Finally, the half-life of a drug has an important bearing on the selection of the most appropriate dosage interval for maintenance therapy. Two situations illustrate this:

(1) If the dosage interval is much longer than the half-life, all drug is effectively eliminated before the next dose, and each dose then represents a new single dose. There is no opportunity for an input–output balance to be achieved and peak concentrations are determined largely by the volume of distribution.

(2) If the dosage interval is much shorter than the half-life, a true steady state is achieved with very minimal plasma level fluctuations. These are determined largely by clearance.

Therefore, depending on the clinical condition and the relationship between blood concentrations and therapeutic effect, dosage schedules can be manipulated to achieve a desired response in individuals if basic pharmacokinetic information such as clearance, volume of distribution and half-life are available.

5.3 INTERPRETATION OF PLASMA LEVELS

Whenever a plasma concentration is measured, it is essential to determine whether or not it is representative of a true steady state. If it is and the drug follows linear pharmacokinetics, the equations outlined above can be used to determine clearance, or it can be used to adjust the dose by simple proportionality.

Clinical example: A 68-year-old man with atrial fibrillation is taking 0.25 mg digoxin daily. Anorexia and nausea have developed and toxicity is suspected. The trough concentration is 2.6 ng/ml: the dose is therefore too high. What should it be ideally?

Assume that 80% of the dose is actually absorbed
$$F = 0.8$$
It is known that the drug is being given once daily
$$\tau = 24 \text{ hours}$$
A trough level is measured at
$$2.6 \text{ ng/ml}$$
Estimate $\overline{Cp_{ss}}$ as
$$2.8 \text{ ng/ml}$$
Therefore
$$Cl = \frac{0.8 \times 250}{2.8 \times 24}$$
$$= 3.0 \text{ l/h or } 50 \text{ ml/min.}$$

A reasonable target $\overline{Cp_{ss}}$ would be 1.5 ng/ml. Therefore, rearranging the clearance equation for dose:

$$\text{Dose} = \frac{Cl \cdot \overline{Cp_{ss}} \cdot \tau}{F}$$

$$= \frac{3.0 \times 1.5 \times 24}{0.8}$$

$$= 0.135 \text{ mg daily}$$

Because of the limitations imposed by commercially available tablets, the choice is 0.125 mg daily, which would produce a $\overline{Cp_{ss}}$ value of 1.4 ng/ml.

Alternatively, the new dose can be quickly arrived at by multiplying the incorrect dose by the ratio of the desired concentration to that observed. Thus

$$\text{Dose} = 0.25 \times \frac{1.5}{2.8} \text{ mg daily}$$

which would lead to the same choice as above, i.e. 0.125 mg daily.

These equations only apply if steady state really exists, and it should be clear that any request for a concentration measurement should be accompanied by *accurate* information. The minimum usually required consists of the following:

(1) *Reason for the request.*

(2) *Time of sample collection* with respect to the previous dose: this helps to estimate Cp_{ss}.

(3) *Drug dose, frequency and route of administration.*

(4) *Duration of therapy*, to assess whether or not steady state has been achieved.

(5) *Relevant patient details* such as age, sex, height, weight and serum creatinine or other index of renal function.

Ideal sampling times, average times to steady state and accepted therapeutic ranges for ten drugs routinely monitored are shown in Table 5.1.

Non steady-state concentration data cannot be treated in this way, and if estimates of pharmacokinetic parameters are required from such data, much more sophisticated analytical techniques are required, with the assistance of computers. It is also essential to remember that drugs showing nonlinear pharmacokinetics cannot be treated in this way and again, resort has to be made to more

TABLE 5.1 Therapeutic ranges and optimal sampling times

Drug	Optimal sampling time	Average time to steady state*	Accepted therapeutic range
Digoxin	5–12 h after dosage	7 days	1–2 ng/ml 1.3–2.6 nmol/l
Disopyramide	(1) During continuous i.v. infusion (2) Immediately before an oral dose	2 days	2–5 µg/ml
Lignocaine	During continuous i.v. infusion	12 hours	2–5 µg/ml
Carbamazepine	Immediately before an oral dose	5 days	4–12 µg/ml 20–50 µmol/l
Phenobarbitone	Unspecific	20 days	10–30 µg/ml 100–150 µmol/l
Phenytoin	Unspecific	14 days	10–20 µg/ml 40–80 µmol/l
Valproic acid	Immediately before an oral dose	3 days	50–100 µg/ml 350–700 µmol/l
Gentamicin	Trough level: immediately before the next dose	3 days	Trough: < 2 µg/ml
Tobramycin	Peak level: 1 h after i.v. or i.m. administration	1 day	Peak: 5–12 µg/ml
Theophylline	Immediately before an oral dose	2 days	10–25 µg/ml

* This assumes the absence of a loading dose.

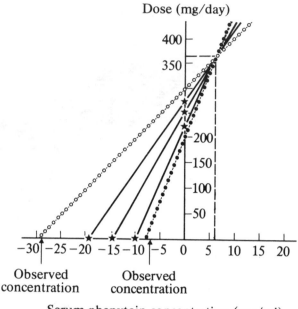

FIG. 5.4 A nomogram for the adjustment of phenytoin dosage which uses steady-state phenytoin concentrations. Two lines are drawn connecting the two phenytoin doses with their respective Cp_{ss} results. These lines are extrapolated to the right of the vertical axis until they intersect. A third line is drawn connecting the point of intersection with the desired Cp_{ss}. The point at which this line cuts the vertical axis is a prediction of the required daily phenytoin dosage for the individual.

sophisticated techniques. In the case of phenytoin, nomograms which relate steady-state concentrations to daily doses are available. An example is shown in Fig. 5.4.

Computer programs

Many computer programs have been devised which aid the interpretation of drug levels in plasma. The most useful ones make estimates of relevant pharmacokinetic parameters such as clearance and volume of distribution in individual patients. Once these estimates have been made, the parameters can then be used to calculate drug doses for any specified steady-state concentration profile.

Programs have now been written which can estimate kinetic parameters from one or two concentration measurements. Initial estimates for the parameters can be obtained from nomograms that

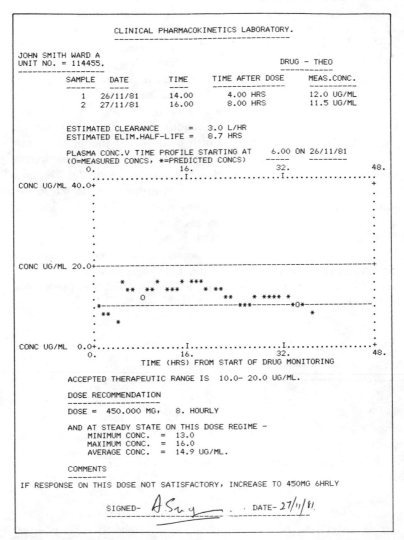

FIG. 5.5   An example of the output from a computer program used in a clinical pharmacokinetics laboratory.

take into account many of the factors listed earlier, for example age, sex, weight, smoking habits, specific diseases, etc. The initial estimates represent typical or average values in the group of patients to which the individual belongs. Information from a plasma concentration, unique to the individual, is then used to revise the initial estimates so that values are produced which are much more representative of that particular individual. Feedback of another concentration measurement can then be used to refine the values even further. This revision procedure is based on statistical probability theory (Bayes Theorem).

An example of the output from such a program is shown in Fig. 5.5. The patient, a male aged 40, had been admitted to hospital with an acute exacerbation of chronic bronchitis. He had been given two 500 mg intravenous injections of aminophylline, 4 hours apart, followed by three 450 mg oral doses of theophylline and blood samples had been taken at the times shown. Theophylline concentrations were 12.0 μg/ml immediately before the first oral dose and 11.5 μg/ml 8 hours after the third oral dose. From this information, and from other details about the patient, i.e. age, weight, smoking habits, etc., clearance was estimated to be 3.0 l/h. Not shown on this report are the estimates for volume of distribution, 37 l and the rate of absorption, 0.35 h^{-1}. These parameter estimates were then used to select a dosage regime that would achieve safe and effective levels, wholly within the therapeutic range.

Cardiac arrhythmias

The use of continuous electrocardiographic monitoring has emphasised the high incidence of arrhythmias occurring not only in patients with cardiac disease but also in otherwise normal subjects. Although an increasing number of drugs with antiarrhythmic activity have become available, many simple arrhythmias do not require treatment. However, there are a number of circumstances in which the indications for treatment are clear:

(1) When the electrophysiological abnormality is life-threatening, e.g. ventricular tachycardia.

(2) When there are major haemodynamic sequelae with hypotension or cardiac failure.

(3) When the patient is markedly symptomatic, e.g. supraventricular tachycardia.

(4) When a simple arrhythmia may lead on to one which is more serious or potentially life-threatening, e.g. warning arrhythmias after acute myocardial infarction.

The choice of the most appropriate antiarrhythmic depends on:

(1) Electrocardiographic diagnosis,

(2) Possible mechanism of the arrhythmia,
(3) Mechanism of action of the drug,
(4) Range of antiarrhythmic activity,
(5) Pharmacokinetic behaviour of the drug,
(6) Haemodynamic effects of the drug.

The aim is to improve cardiovascular function either by cardioversion to sinus rhythm or by conversion to a more desirable pattern of electrical and mechanical activity.

6.1   RELEVANT PATHOPHYSIOLOGY

Normal electrophysiology

For the purposes of understanding its electrophysiology, cardiac tissue can be divided into two types.

(1) Ordinary muscle, which constitutes most of the atria and ventricles.

(2) Specialised conducting tissue, e.g. the sinoatrial (SA) and antrioventricular (AV) nodes and His Parkinje system.

In the ordinary muscle depolarisation is very rapid and is the result of sodium channels in the membrane opening and allowing sodium to pass down its electrochemical gradient. This is referred to as phase 0 of the action potential (Fig. 6.1). It is followed by a slower phase of repolarisation. In contrast, the specialised tissue action potential is characterised by slow depolarisation which depends largely on 'slow channel' calcium currents (Phase 4, Fig. 6.1). These tissues also possess the property of automaticity, i.e. spontaneous depolarisation and impulse formation. Automaticity is physiological in specialised tissues, but pathological elsewhere in the myocardium.

Mechanisms of arrhythmias

Abnormal automaticity or impaired conduction form the basis of most arrhythmias. Automaticity may be pathologically increased in specialised tissue, or appear in ordinary tissue because of ischaemia, electrolyte disturbance, acidosis or drug effects, e.g. digoxin toxicity. The result can be repetitive depolarisation and impulse propagation.

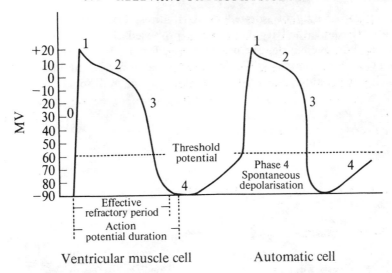

FIG. 6.1 Schematic representation of an action potential measured in a ventricular muscle cell and in a specialised cell demonstrating automaticity.

Under normal conditions the rate of impulse conduction is reduced by the slow current depolarisation of the AV node. Ischaemia can enhance this slowing and lead to various degrees of conduction block. Alternatively, ischaemia, electrolyte disturbance, etc. can result in cells changing from rapid to slow depolarisation. In either case, the resulting conduction block favours the establishment of re-entry arrhythmias. This occurs when an impulse deviates from a pathway of slowed conduction towards adjacent myocardium which is no longer refractory. Excitation of cardiac tissue with, for example, coupled ventricular beats or sustained ventricular tachycardia can occur.

Classification of antiarrhythmic drugs

Antiarrhythmic agents can be categorised in a practical sense according to their anatomical site of action. Some act predominantly on *ventricular* arrhythmias, e.g. lignocaine. Others have an *atrial* action, e.g. verapamil, and some have an action on both atria and ventricles, e.g. disopyramide. An alternative theoretical classification in widespread use was proposed by Vaughan Williams and Singh following observations on the electrical activity of isolated cardiac fibres. Four types of basic antiarrhythmic activity have been proposed. Some drugs have more than one action, but in clinically effective dosage, one action generally predominates (Table 6.1). The action of digitalis is not included in this classification, and is considered separately on p. 68.

TABLE 6.1   Classifications of antiarrhythmic drugs

Class	Drugs
I. Membrane-stabilising agents	A. Quinidine-like agents. Procainamide, disopyramide, Lorcainide, Encainide (both under investigation)
	B. Lignocaine, phenytoin, mexiletine, tocainide.
	C. Aprinidine (under investigation)
II. Antisympathetic agents	Beta blockers. Bretylium (also Class III activity)
III. Agents widening action potential duration	Amiodarone. Sotalol (also beta blocker)
IV. Calcium antagonists	Verapamil

Class I action: membrane stabilising activity and interference with depolarisation of the cardiac cell membrane by restricting the entry of the depolarising fast sodium current. Some of these agents have differing activity when their effects are studied with His bundle recordings, and they can be further subdivided on this basis (Table 6.1).

Class II action: decrease arrhythmogenic effects of catecholamines. Beta adrenoceptor blocking compounds act as competitive antagonists. Bretylium blocks the release of sympathetic transmitter and has a similar antiarrhythmic effect, and may also have class III activity.

Class III action: prolongs the duration of the action potential of atrial and ventricular muscle with associated prolongation of the effective refractory period.

Class IV action: results from inhibition of the slow inward Ca^{++} mediated current. This action is of importance in the upper and middle nodal regions and may have particular value in blocking one limb of a re-entry circuit.

6.2   CLASS IA AGENTS

Quinidine

Mechanism

Quinidine reduces the maximal rate of depolarisation, depresses spontaneous phase 4 diastolic depolarisation in automatic cells, slows conduction and prolongs the effective refractory period of atrial, ventricular and Purkinje fibres.

Pharmacokinetics

Seventy per cent of the drug is absorbed from the gut. With conventional preparations measurable levels are obtained within 15 min and the peak effect occurs between 1–3 h. However, because the average half-life is of the order of 6 h, slow-release preparations are more commonly used. It is 80–90% bound to plasma proteins and is metabolised by hydroxylation; the inactive metabolites are excreted in the urine. Antiarrhythmic effects are seen with drug levels of 2.3–5 $\mu g/ml$.

Adverse effects

Higher concentrations are associated with decreased myocardial contractility: peripheral vasodilation and hypotension; electrophysiological effects with possible sinus arrest or sinoatrial block, progressive QRS and QT prolongation, which may lead to paroxysmal ventricular tachycardia with torsade despointes. Toxic concentrations may also lead to AV dissociation. Other adverse effects include gastrointestinal symptoms with nausea, vomiting, diarrhoea; cinchonism; and hypersensitivity reactions with fever, purpura, thrombocytopaenia and hepatic dysfunction. In cirrhosis the clearance of quinidine is reduced. There is also less binding to plasma proteins and hence lower plasma levels are effective (p. 14). Quinidine has a vagolytic action which increases AV conduction. This may lead to rapid conduction from atrial to ventricles. In the treatment of atrial tachycardia or atrial flutter, digitalis should be given prior to quinidine administration.

Drug interactions

Quinidine interacts with digoxin and may precipitate digoxin toxicity. Digoxin plasma levels are increased and the dose of digoxin must be reduced to compensate for this.

Clinical use and dose

Quinidine now has limited clinical use, e.g. prophylaxis following cardioversion. The dose is 200–600 mg orally 6 hourly after initial test dose.

Procainamide

Mechanism

Similar electrophysiological properties to quinidine with typical class I activity but also shown experimentally that ventricular fibrillation threshold is increased.

Pharmacokinetics

Procainamide can be administered orally being 75% bioavailable. Again, because it has a relatively short half-life of the order of 3.5 h, it is usually given as a slow-release preparation. The compound is metabolised to N-acetyl procainamide (NAPA), which has antiarrhythmic activity in its own right. Antiarrhythmic activity of procainamide occurs at blood levels of 4–10 μg/ml, and toxic effects are likely with blood levels of 16 μg/ml. Relatively high plasma levels of both parent drug and NAPA occur in renal impairment and cardiac failure.

The drug is metabolised by acetylation in the liver. The enzyme, which is bimodally distributed in the population, also metabolises isoniazid and hydralazine; slow acetylators theoretically require smaller doses for antiarrhythmic activity than fast acetylators.

Adverse effects

These may follow rapid intravenous administration and include hypotension with vasodilatation and reduced cardiac output. ECG changes include QRS and QT prolongation. In higher doses PR prolongation may occur with delayed AV conduction leading to heart block. On chronic oral therapy at high dosage many patients develop a drug-induced lupus erythematosus syndrome with positive anti-nuclear factors. However, there is usually absence of renal effects. This is particularly common in slow acetylators.

Drug interactions

Procainamide reduces the antimicrobial effect of sulphonamides. The mechanism appears to be formation of para-aminobenzoic acid from procaine.

Clinical use and dose

It is useful in the full spectrum of arrhythmias arising from atrial, junctional and ventricular tissue, including lignocaine-resistant ventricular rhythms. Administered intravenously, 50–100 mg every 5 minutes to a total dose of 1000 mg. Oral dosage is 250–500 mg 3 hourly orally or by slow-release preparation.

Disopyramide

Mechanism

Disopyramide has electrophysiological properties similar to quinidine.

Pharmacokinetics

Disopyramide is 70–80% bioavailable. The half-life in normal subjects is 6–8 h. Fifty per cent is excreted unchanged in the urine; a further 25% is excreted in the form of the main metabolite: the *N*-dealkylated form of disopyramide. The dose should be reduced in severe renal failure when creatinine clearance levels are less than 25 ml/min. The therapeutic range is 2–5 μg/ml.

Adverse effects

These are related primarily to anticholinergic activity with urinary retention, glaucoma and blurred vision. QT prolongation occurs with increasing plasma concentrations, and this may also predispose to re-entry arrhythmias. Relative contraindications to therapy include sick sinus syndrome, prostate hypertrophy and cardiac failure.

Drug interactions

Disopyramide enhances the negative effects of quinidine or digoxin on the conducting system.

Clinical use and dose

Atrial and ventricular arrhythmias including those resistant to lignocaine. The dose is 100–200 mg 6 hourly orally. Also available for slow intravenous injection, 2 mg/kg.

CLASS 1B AGENTS

Lignocaine

Mechanism

Lignocaine has local anaesthetic activity and typical class I anti-arrhythmic activity. The conduction velocity in Purkinje fibres and in ventricular muscle is only marginally slowed. Lignocaine is the standard agent in ventricular arrhythmias following myocardial infarction and cardiac surgery.

Pharmacokinetics

Lignocaine is not given orally because it is hydrolysed in the gastrointestinal tract and is submitted to extensive first-pass metabolism in the liver so that adequate blood levels are not achieved. Following intravenous administration, elimination half-life is about

100 min. The clearance of lignocaine is reduced in cardiac failure and lower rates of infusion are required (p. 21).

Adverse effects

Although therapeutic concentrations have little haemodynamic effect, high levels of lignocaine cause bradycardia, hypotension and even asystole. Gastrointestinal symptoms with nausea and vomiting may also occur. At levels higher than 5 μg/ml central nervous system adverse effects may occur with paraesthesiae, twitching and even grand mal seizures.

Clinical use and dose

Lignocaine has no action on atrial arrhythmias, but it is particularly useful in ventricular arrhythmias after myocardial infarction including R on T or multifocal ventricular extrasystoles or episodes of ventricular tachycardia. Although the intramuscular route has been advocated in domiciliary practice, absorption tends to be erratic and blood levels achieved vary widely according to the haemodynamic status of the patient. Therefore, lignocaine is routinely given by the intravenous route. 1–2 mg/kg body weight is given by rapid injection followed by an infusion of 2 mg/min to maintain arrhythmia suppression. Therapeutic blood levels are 1.5–5 μg/ml.

Tocainide

Tocainide is a lignocaine analogue that is active after both intravenous and oral administration. Its haemodynamic and electroplysiological actions are similar to lignocaine, and its potential use is as an alternative to this standard agent with the advantage of long-term oral administration.

Dose

The dose is 500–750 mg i.v. over 30 min followed by 600–800 mg orally. The maintenance dose is 1200–2400 mg daily in divided doses.

Mexiletine

Mechanism

This primary amine has similar electrophysiological action to lignocaine.

Pharmacokinetics

It is active after both oral and intravenous administration. It is extensively metabolised to parahydroxy- and hydroxy-methyl-mexiletine and to their corresponding deaminated alcohols by hepatic metabolism. The half-life in normal subjects is 9–12 h. However, this may be increased, particularly following acute myocardial infarction. Oral absorption is reduced when given with morphine or diamorphine.

Adverse effects

Toxic effects include nausea, dizziness, drowsiness, tremor and hypotension and are common at plasma levels above 2.0 μg/ml.

Clinical use and dose

Mexiletine is used in the treatment of ventricular arrhythmias and is particularly useful as an alternative to lignocaine. Mexiletine is given initially intravenously by bolus injection, 1–3 mg/kg then 20–45 μg/kg/min by intravenous infusion, followed by 0.6–1.2 g orally in 24 h. Effective plasma levels are 0.75–2.0 μg/ml; the therapeutic range is narrow.

Phenytoin

Phenytoin has class I activity but in addition in hypokalaemiait reduces the duration of the action potential in Purkinje and ventricular fibres. Haemodynamic adverse effects include dose-related impairment of myocardial contractility following intravenous use. Adverse effects are reviewed on p. 270. In clinical use as an alternative to lignocaine or in digoxin-induced arrhythmias phenytoin is given by 50–100 mg rapid doses over 5 min up to 1000 mg.

6.3 CLASS II AGENTS

Beta-adrenoceptor antagonists

The pharmacokinetics, adverse effects and mechanisms of action are discussed in Chapter 8.3.

Clinical use

These compounds are particularly useful for the control of inappropriate sinus tachycardia or supraventricular arrhythmias provoked by conditions of high catecholamine excretion including emotion, exercise or anaesthesia. For intravenous use most experience has been gained using practolol although metoprolol, propranolol and acebutolol have all been used. Beta adrenoceptor blockers are also useful in the control of ventricular arrhythmias associated with a fast sinus rate in the absence of cardiac failure. Their prophylactic use in the reduction of sudden death after myocardial infarction has been suggested and recent studies with timolol, propranolol, alprenolol, metoprolol and atenolol have been encouraging. Other clinical situations in which the beta blockers are useful include mitral valve prolapse, hypertrophic obstructive cardiomyopathy and hereditary prolonged QT syndrome.

Bretylium tosylate

This has adrenergic neurone blocking activity and suppresses noradrenaline release. It is eliminated by the kidney with a half-life of 7–12 hours. Bretylium also has class III action of Purkinje fibres and is effective in ventricular arrhythmias, particularly ventricular fibrillation refractory to lignocaine or procainamide and repeated electrical defibrillation.

Adverse effects include hypotension.

It is administered by the intravenous route, 5–10 mg/kg or intramuscular route 5 mg/kg.

6.4 CLASS III AGENTS

Amiodarone

Mechanism

Prolongation of action potential duration and increased refractory period. In addition it may have some beta receptor blocking activity and a quinidine-like effect at higher dose.

Pharmacokinetics

After oral administration, amiodarone is very slowly eliminated with an effective half-life of over 30 days. There is no relationship between the plasma level and antiarrhythmic activity; considerable accumulation occurs in muscle and fat. The therapeutic effect develops over several days.

Adverse effects

Amiodarone has little haemodynamic effect and has little electrophysiological toxicity, except that it may depress sinus node automaticity and conduction at the atrioventricular node level. Amiodarone is contraindicated if intraventricular or AV block is present. The compound contains iodine and may interfere with thyroid function, causing hypo- or hyperthyroidism. Corneal micro deposits occur with use of this agent; they are reversible and can be diminished by withdrawing therapy or using sodium–iodine heparinate eye drops. Photosensitisation occurs in 10% of patients. Gastrointestinal adverse effects are also relatively common.

Clinical use and dose

Amiodarone has been shown to be of value in a wide range of ventricular and supraventricular arrhythmias. It is particularly useful with Wolff–Parkinson–White syndrome by inhibiting supraventricular resistant tachycardias by an action on both anomalous and normal pathways of conduction. At present drug usage is limited to arrhythmias refractory to the usual first line agents. Amiodarone is given orally 300–600 mg daily; the use of the intravenous preparation remains under study.

6.5 CLASS IV AGENTS

Verapamil

Mechanism

Electrophysiological activity is to inhibit slow inward Ca^{++} mediated current. It decreases AV conduction.

Pharmacokinetics

Bioavailability is 10–20%. It is eliminated by the kidneys.

Adverse effects

Contraindicated in heart block. Caution must also be observed where significant myocardial disease is present. Additional effects include nausea, dizziness, and facial flushing. In SA node dysfunction sinus bradycardia, sinus arrest, hypotension and even asystole may occur.

Drug interactions

Potentiates the negative effect of digoxin on AV conduction and also enhances the negative inotropic effects of beta blockers.

Clinical use and dose

Verapamil is particularly useful in re-entry supraventricular arrhythmias by inhibiting one limb of the re-entry circuit. Increased AV block also allows control of the ventricular rate in atrial flutter and atrial fibrillation. Mainly useful in supraventicular arrhythmias; there is little action on ventricular arrhythmias. Verapamil can be used by both oral and intravenous routes. Oral verapamil takes 2–4 hours to act with peak effect at 5 h; therapeutic levels 100–200 µg/ml. Intravenous dosing shows haemodynamic effects peaking at 5 min and of 20 min duration. AV node action occurs at 10–15 min and lasts 6 h suggesting binding at the nodal tract. Intravenous verapamil is administered by infusion or rapid injection, 5–10 mg with infusion rates of 0.005 mg/kg/min. Oral dosage is 40–120 mg thrice daily.

6.6 DIGITALIS GLYCOSIDES

The term digitalis or digitalis glycoside refers to any of the cardioactive steroids which share an aglycone ring structure and have positive inotropic and electrophysiological effects.

Mechanism

A major effect is to decrease sodium transport out of the cardiac cell by inhibiting Na^+/K^+ ATPase (the sodium pump). The resulting accumulation of sodium results in a poorly understood increase of intracellular calcium ions which is probably responsible for the positive inotropic effects of digitalis glycosides. In addition, the actions of these drugs at the membrane result in even less well understood electrophysiological changes which decrease cardiac conduction at the AV node and bundle of His and sensitise the sinoatrial node to vagal impulses. At high concentrations, digitalis glycosides increase myocardial automaticity, possibly because inhibition of the sodium pump leads to a decrease of membrane resting potential towards threshold.

The three major effects of digitalis glycosides on the heart are thus:

(1) Positive inotropic effect.

(2) Decreased ventricular rate in atrial fibrillation or flutter, by decreasing AV conduction.

(3) Increased myocardial automaticity in high (toxic) concentrations, or at 'therapeutic' concentrations if other factors such as hypokalaemia are present.

Pharmacockinetics

Digoxin can be given orally or intravenously. The average volume of distribution is approximately 7.3 l/kg; this is decreased in patients with renal disease, hypothyroidism and in patients taking quinidine. It is increased in thyrotoxicosis. Clearance varies from individual to individual and is the result of both renal and metabolic elimination mechanisms. In healthy adults, the metabolic component is of the order of 40–60 ml/min/70 kg, and the renal component approximates creatinine clearance. Metabolic clearance is reduced in congestive cardiac failure. Clearance in any individual can be calculated by the equations discussed in Chapter 5.3.

In patients with normal renal function, the elimination half-life is approximately 2 days. In patients with severe renal disease, the half-life increases to approximately 4–6 days.

Digitoxin is more lipid soluble than digoxin and is practically 100% absorbed from the gastrointestinal tract. It is given orally and intravenously. It is extensively metabolised by the liver, and the elimination half-life is 5–7 days. Renal impairment does not appreciably alter digitoxin kinetics but binding to plasma proteins, normally of the order of 90–97%, may be slightly decreased in uraemia.

It seems likely that digitoxin is excreted in the bile and is then reabsorbed to some extent, i.e. it has an enterohepatic circulation. Cholestyramine, which can bind cardiac glycosides in the gut, can interrupt the enterohepatic circulation; whether it can shorten the duration of digitoxin toxicity is still a matter for speculation.

Ouabain is poorly absorbed from the gut and is administered exclusively by the intravenous route. Its onset of action is rapid, and it has a somewhat shorter half-life than digoxin: approximately 1 day. Elimination is mainly renal.

Adverse effects

Determined in part by plasma concentration (> 2.5 ng/ml for digoxin) and in part by electrolyte balance. Digoxin and potassium compete for cardiac receptor sites and hypokalaemia can precipitate digitalis adverse effects. Hypercalcaemia also potentiates toxicity.

The common extracardiac adverse effects are:

Anorexia, nausea and vomiting,

Fatigue,

Weakness,

Diarrhoea.

Less commonly, neurological symptoms including difficulty in reading, confusion or even psychosis can occur. Abdominal pain is another less common manifestation.

The cardiac adverse effects are:

Premature ventricular ectopic beats or ventricular fibrillation,

Junctional rhythm,

Various degrees of AV block, including complete heart block,

Atrial or ventricular tachycardia,
Sinus bradycardia or sinus arrest.

Cardiac signs precede extracardiac in about 50% of cases. A common effect of digitalis glycosides on the ECG, prolonged P–R interval and ST segments depression, does *not* indicate toxicity.

Drug interactions

Digoxin absorption is decreased by drugs that increase intestinal motility, e.g. metoclopramide, and increased by drugs such as propantheline that decrease motility. Many antacids, particularly magnesium trisilicate, reduce digoxin absorption. Digoxin levels increase if quinidine is co-administered and toxicity can occur. The potential for toxicity is enhanced for all cardiac glycosides when diuretics are co-administered because of hypokalaemia.

Clinical use and doses

The principal indication for the use of cardiac glycosides in congestive heart failure *associated with* atrial fibrillation and inappropriately rapid ventricular rate. The beneficial effects result mainly from the reduction in frequency of ventricular response, secondary to the depression of AV conduction. This effect is in addition to, and probably more important than, the inotropic action. The indication for cardiac glycosides in cardiac failure with sinus rhythm is less clear. The availability of potent diuretics make them the first line treatment. In high output states such as thyrotoxicosis and in pulmonary heart disease the response to digoxin in patients with sinus rhythm is disappointing.

All glycosides share the genin or aglycone ring structure combined with one to four molecules of sugar which modify the compound's properties. The choice of agent depends on:

(1) Route of administration required,
(2) Desired speed of action,
(3) Duration of action required.

The drugs most used in clinical practice are digoxin, digitoxin and ouabain.

The dosing schedules used with the cardiac glycosides depend not only on the pharmacokinetic properties of the drug but also on factors that determine individual susceptibility. The general approach is usually to introduce a loading dose of the glycoside and then to follow this by a maintenance dose. The loading dose is determined by the volume of distribution and the desired plasma concentration the maintenance dose by clearance (Chapter 5). If a maintenance dose is employed without a loading dose, drug accumulation and activity develop slowly because steady state is not reached for 4 to 5 half-lives. With digoxin the major determinant of clearance is renal function and the maintenance dose for this glycoside must be reduced if renal function is subnormal and excretion is impaired. Nomograms and simple equations can be used to estimate the most appropriate loading and maintenance doses. However, these must remain approximations and the patient's clinical response must influence long-term management. Standard loading and maintenance doses of the glycosides are shown in Table 6.2.

TABLE 6.2 Loading and maintenance doses of glycosides

Drug	Average loading dose		Usual daily oral maintenance dose (normal renal function)
	Oral	i.v.	
Ouabain		0.3–0.5 mg	—
Digoxin	1.0–1.5 mg	0.3–1.0 mg	0.125–0.25 mg
Digitoxin	1.05 mg	1.0 mg	0.1 mg

The use of drug monitoring of the plasma levels of the glycosides has been useful, particularly to monitor digoxin levels in renal impairment and toxicity. The normal therapeutic range of digoxin is 1–2 ng/ml. Venous sampling should be performed 3–4 h after an i.v. dose or 6–8 h after an oral dose. If blood levels are low then compliance should be checked, possible causes of malabsorption considered and, in the case of digitoxin, causes of interruption of the enterohepatic circulation or increased hepatic metabolism should be considered.

Treatment of digitalis induced toxicity

Treatment of digitalis induced arrhythmias is often difficult. The glycoside should be withdrawn, and if hypokalaemia is present, potassium chloride should be administered by infusion at a rate of 20 mmol/h (not exceeding 100 mmol total) with electrocardiographic and biochemical monitoring.

Ventricular arrhythmias may require lignocaine or phenytoin administration. Supraventricular arrhythmias may respond to beta blockade or phenytoin. Care must be observed using verapamil and procainamide as increased degrees of heat block may occur. Temporary pacing may be required for heart block with haemodynamic effects or in the rare instance of S A node arrest.

CHAPTER 7

Heart failure and angina pectoris

7.1 Heart failure

7.2 Angina pectoris

7.1 HEART FAILURE

Aims

Improve cardiac performance; reduce symptoms caused by pulmonary venous congestion and peripheral oedema.

Relevant pathophysiology

Cardiac performance is determined by:

(1) *Preload:* ventricular end-diastolic pressure and volume. A clinically relevant increase of preload results from:
  (a) Increased venous return,
  (b) Increased total blood volume.
In normal hearts an increased preload leads to increased end-diastolic fibre length which in turn causes increased force of contraction. In heart failure this response is reduced or even reversed.

(2) *Force of cardiac contraction:* determined largely by the intrinsic strength and integrity of the muscle cells.

Force of contraction is decreased by:
   (a) Myocardial ischaemia,
   (b) Myocardial infarction,
   (c) Rhythm disturbance.

(3) *Afterload:* ventricular wall tension developed during ejection. Afterload is increased by:
   (a) Increased aortic pressure,
   (b) Increased ventricular cavity size.

Heart failure exists when cardiac output is insufficient to meet the requirements of tissue perfusion. In Western countries heart failure is usually caused by one of the following:
   (1) Myocardial ischaemia,
   (2) Myocardial infarction,
   (3) Hypertension leading to ventricular hypertrophy (Chapter 8),
   (4) Arrhythmias (Chapter 6).

In response to heart failure, *compensatory mechanisms* are activated:
   (1) Sodium and water retention; this has beneficial and adverse consequences:
      (a) *Beneficial:* improves perfusion by increasing intravascular volume.
      (b) *Adverse:* increases preload. In the failing heart the beneficial limits of increasing myocardial fibre length are eventually exceeded. Pulmonary congestion and peripheral oedema develop.
   (2) Increased activity of adrenergic nervous system; this also has beneficial and adverse aspects.
      (a) *Beneficial:* increased myocardial contractility; maintains cardiac output and blood pressure.
      (b) *Adverse:* increased afterload and, therefore, myocardial oxygen demand; increased peripheral vascular resistance may reduce tissue perfusion; tachyarrhythmias.

DRUGS USED IN HEART FAILURE

(1) *Diuretics:* thiazides, loop diuretics:
   (a) Decrease peripheral and pulmonary oedema,
   (b) Decrease preload by reduction in circulatory volume.

(2) *Drugs that have a positive inotropic effect:* cardiac glycosides; beta adrenoceptor agonists.

(3) *Drugs that off load the ventricles:*

(a) Mainly decrease preload: glyceryl trinitrate, isosorbide dinitrate,

(b) Mainly decrease afterload: hydralazine; captopril,

(c) Decrease both preload and afterload: sodium nitroprusside; prazosin.

Diuretics

These drugs are first-line treatment for patients with heart failure. In mild failure a thiazide diuretic may suffice (p. 100). Moderate or severe failure requires a loop diuretic.

Loop diuretics: Frusemide, bumetanide, ethacrynic acid

Mechanism

Primarily inhibition of Na^+/K^+ ATPase in the ascending limb of loop of Henle with increased salt and water loss. The increased delivery of sodium to distal tubule encourages Na^+/K^+ exchange with a tendency to a hypokalaemic alkalosis.

Pharmacokinetics

All three drugs are well absorbed following oral administration and are also available in intravenous formulations. Elimination is largely by renal excretion with a small contribution by liver metabolism. These drugs have a rapid onset and short duration of action.

Adverse effects

Salt and water depletion can occur; not so much an adverse reaction as excessive use of these powerful drugs. Potassium depletion of clinical importance occurs more often than with thiazides; regular monitoring of potassium is required and additional potassium supplementation advisable. Glucose intolerance and urate retention can occur as with thiazides. Rapid intravenous injection of large doses can produce deafness.

Drug interactions

These include potentiation of nephrotoxic effects of gentamicin and cephaloridine; hypokalaemia enhances the risk of digoxin toxicity.

Dose

Frusemide: Oral: 20 mg each morning up to 1 or 2 g each day in very resistant oedema or cardiac failure.

Intravenous: 20–40 mg slowly. In resistant cases up to 1 g can be infused over 2–4 hours.

Bumetanide: Oral: 0.5–5 mg each day.

Intravenous: 0.5–2 mg or infusion up to 5 mg slowly.

Ethacrynic acid: Oral: 25–150 mg daily.

Intravenous: slow infusion of 50 mg.

Potassium supplementation

There are three occasions where supplementation of dietary potassium is likely to be required:

(1) Administration of high doses of loop diuretics in treating heart failure.

(2) Co-administration of digoxin, since hypokalaemia potentiates digoxin toxicity.

(3) Administration of a thiazide diuretic to a patient with a poor potassium intake, e.g. the older patient.

In general, a serum potassium below 3.5 mmol/l is a definite indication for potassium supplements in a patient receiving digoxin and a relative indication in others.

Potassium supplements are available as the chloride salt in tablets of 8 or 12 mmol and granules of 20 mmol. Starting dose from 8 mmol two or three times daily.

Potassium sparing diuretics

As an alternative to giving potassium it is possible to give drugs that decrease potassium excretion. These drugs are all diuretics themselves, but their effect is weak and they are rarely used alone.

(1) **Amiloride:** decreases potassium loss caused by loop diuretics and thiazides.

Dose: 5–20 mg daily.

(2) **Triamterene:** as for amiloride.
Dose: 100–200 mg/day.

(3) **Spironolactone:** competitively inhibits the effects of aldosterone. It is, therefore, useful in treating the oedema of conditions associated with excess aldosterone: cirrhosis and refractory heart failure. In addition, it is effective in high doses for the treatment of the rare condition of primary aldosteronism (Conn's syndrome).

Doses: 100–200 mg/day in divided doses. 300 mg/day for primary aldosteronism.

The adverse effect common to all these drugs is hyperkalaemia, and is particularly likely in patients with inpaired renal function. Potassium supplements must *never* be given together with a potassium sparing diuretic. Spironolactone commonly causes nausea, gynaecomastia in men and menstrual irregularities in women. It can decrease the renal secretion of digoxin.

Comment

Potassium sparing drugs are widely prescribed in proprietary formulations combined with a thiazide. This is quite illogical in view of the infrequent requirements for potassium supplementation in patients receiving thiazides. It is also expensive, combination tablets costing five to ten times more than thiazide alone.

Drugs that have a positive inotropic effect

Digitalis glycosides: Digoxin, Digitoxin.

The pharmacodynamics and pharmacokinetics of digoxin together with clinical uses and doses are discussed in full in Chapter 6.6.

Once considered an indispensable part of anti-failure treatment, the role of digoxin is again questioned. Digoxin improves cardiac performance in patients with tachyarrhythmias. In patients in sinus rhythm, digoxin has a positive inotropic effect when given acutely, but there is considerable doubt as to whether this effect is maintained in long-term therapy. The current balance of evidence is that it is not. In some trials as many as 80% of patients *in sinus rhythm* showed no deterioration when digoxin was stopped.

In view of its toxicity digoxin should not be used in the

long-term treatment of heart failure unless atrial fibrillation is an aetiological factor. If digoxin is used the dose should be adjusted to take account of renal function. Monitoring of plasma drug levels may be useful.

Comment

The controversy relating to digoxin in heart failure with sinus rhythm is not new. During the eighteenth century, Withering in his writings on what we now know to be digitalis, indicated that its role was mainly in oedematous patients with irregular heart rhythms. However, an uncritical approach to therapy has led to extensive use in types of heart failure where benefit is unlikely but the risks of drug treatment remain.

Adrenoceptor agonists: Dopamine, dobutamine and prenalterol

These drugs are currently used only in acute severe heart failure accompanied by hypotension and poor tissue perfusion. They have established short-term effects when given intravenously.

Mechanism

All three drugs produce their inotropic effect by $beta_1$-adrenoceptor stimulation of the myocardium. The effects of dopamine are dose dependent and depend partly on direct action and partly on indirect effects through increased noradrenaline release. Below 5 μg/kg/min the major effect is to increase renal blood flow by stimulation of dopamine receptors. As the dose is increased in the 5–20 μg/kg/min range both $beta_1$- and alpha-adrenoceptor stimulant effects are seen with increased cardiac output and a modest rise in blood pressure. Above this dose range alpha-receptor effects are more marked with a further rise in blood pressure; this tends to increase afterload and is undesirable. Dobutamine has no renal vasodilator effect, less vasoconstrictor (alpha) effect and a similar inotropic effect to dopamine. Prenalterol is a selective $beta_1$-agonist which is under clinical evaluation.

Pharmacokinetics

These drugs undergo rapid clearance. Dopamine and dobutamine must be given intravenously but prenalterol is also available in an oral formulation.

Adverse effects

Mainly tachyarrhythmias from $beta_1$-receptor stimulation when used in excessive doses.

Doses

Dopamine: 5 μg/kg/min initially, increasing as required by the clinical response.
Dobutamine: 2.5 μg/kg/min initially, increasing as necessary.
Prenalterol: dose range under evaluation.

Drugs that offload the ventricles by reducing preload and afterload

Many drugs with vasodilator activity have shown beneficial actions in cardiac failure by reducing aortic impedence (afterload) or reducing cardiac venous return (preload). The usefulness of an individual drug depends on the haemodynamic changes in the individual patient and its relative effect on preload and afterload. Venodilators reduce the left ventricular end diastolic pressure and volume; arteriolar dilators reduce aortic impedance and greatly enhance cardiac output. In Table 7.1 the haemodynamic indications for arterial, venous and mixed vasodilators are shown.

TABLE 7.1   Haemodynamic indications for arterial, venous and mixed vasodilators

Cardiac index	Left ventricular filling pressure	Vasodilator
Adequate (> 2.5L/min/sq. m)	Markedly elevated (> 25 mmHg)	Nitroglycerin, Isosorbide dinitrate
Markedly reduced (< 2.5L/mm/sq. m)	Adequate (14–25 mmHg)	Hydralazine, Captopril
Markedly reduced (< 2.5L/mm/sq. m)	Markedly elevated (> 25 mmHg)	Combination of Hydralazine and Nitrate, Nitroprusside, Prazosin

Vasodilators have been shown to be of value in patients with hypertensive heart disease, endstage ischaemic heart disease, congestive cardiomyopathy and mitral or aortic regurgitation. They are contraindicated in the presence of obstructive or stenotic valvular lesions such as mitral or aortic stenosis.

Drugs affecting preload

Glyceryl trinitrate

Sublingual nitroglycerin leads to direct relaxation of smooth muscle in the systemic venous system. Subsequent venous pooling in cardiac failure leads to a reduction in left ventricular end diastolic pressure and volume reducing pulmonary congestion. There is usually no associated rise in cardiac output.

Intravenous glyceryl trinitrate can be used acutely until oral agents can be introduced.

Long-acting nitrates have been shown to have beneficial long-term haemodynamic effects in heart failure.
Dose: Isosorbide dinitrate 20–40 mg three times daily.

Similar effects have been shown with pentaerythritol tetranitrate, oral-controlled release nitroglycerin and cutaneous nitroglycerin ointment.

Drugs affecting afterload

Hydralazine

This has a direct vasodilator effect confined to the arterial bed. Reduction in systemic vascular resistance leads to a considerable rise of cardiac output. Changes in arterial blood pressure and heart rate are very small in patients with heart failure.
Dose: up to 200 mg daily in divided doses.

Captopril

The antihypertensive agent that inhibits angiotensin-converting enzyme and prevents the formation of angiotensin II (p. 107), has also been found acutely and chronically to improve cardiac performance and symptoms in chronic heart failure. The actions on arteriolar resistance are well established but captopril may also have some venous effects.

Dose: 25–75 mg twice or three times daily, increasing if necessary.

Drugs with effects on preload and afterload

Sodium nitroprusside

This is a mixed venous and arteriolar dilator also used for acute reduction of blood pressure (p. 92). It must be given intravenously by continuous infusion in a dose range 25–125 μg/min. Blood pressure falls rapidly and the effect wears off over 1–2 min after stopping the infusion. This agent is particularly useful in acute cardiac failure following myocardial infarction and in acute valvular insufficiency, such as mitral incompetence following acute infarct or aortic incompetence in bacterial endocarditis. It should not be used for more than 24–48 hours because of accumulation of thiocyanate.

Prazosin

This is an alpha-1 selective (postsynaptic) receptor antagonist which causes mixed venous and arteriolar dilatation (p. 105). Its haemodynamic profile of action is similar to sodium nitroprusside. It can be administered orally and provides a rational long-term therapy for patients who have shown clinical responses to intravenous sodium nitroprusside. In patients with chronic heart failure it reduces filling pressure and augments cardiac output. Tolerance may develop but this can be overcome by increasing the dose or alternatively stopping therapy for days or weeks with re-introduction of prazosin.

Dose: It is given orally as 1–10 mg in two or three divided doses.

Comment

Vasodilators at present are used in patients with severe cardiac failure with grade III or grade IV (New York Heart Association) symptoms. Further experience may extend their use to milder cases in the future. Choice of drug depends on the haemodynamic findings in the individual patient. If cardiac output is low and filling pressure is moderate then an arteriolar dilator is indicated. If the filling pressure is high and cardiac output adequate, then a venous dilator is indicated. If the filling pressure is high and cardiac output low a mixed dilator is indicated.

Long-acting nitrates and hydralazine can be used together to gain the beneficial haemodynamic effects on preload and afterload respectively.

GENERAL PRINCIPLES OF MANAGEMENT

Acute left ventricular failure or pulmonary oedema presents with severe breathlessness, orthopnoea or nocturnal dyspnoea.
(1) Sit the patient up,
(2) Apply 100% oxygen,
(3) Establish an i.v. line,
(4) Give 5 mg diamorphine or 10 mg morphine i.v. because:
    (a) It has a venodilator effect reducing preload,
    (b) It reduces the intense distress of the patient,
(5) Give frusemide 40 mg i.v., more if the patient is already receiving a loop diuretic, because:
    (a) It has a rapid offloading effect resulting
from venous dilatation,
    (b) It has a slower offloading effect resulting from diuresis and natriuresis,
(6) Give aminophylline 250 mg i.v. slowly over 10–20 min because:
    (a) It has a positive inotropic effect,
    (b) It has a bronchodilating effect,
    (c) It has a modest effect on renal blood flow and may augment the action of the diuretic,
(7) If these measures fail it may be necessary to offload with intravenous sodium nitroprusside.

Cardiogenic shock consists of hypotension and oliguria with clinical signs of poor tissue perfusion. It is usually caused by recent extensive myocardial infarction.
(1) Where possible, monitor both arterial and pulmonary wedge pressure,
(2) Give 100% oxygen,

(3) Try to improve cardiac performance with dopamine or a similar inotropic drug,

(4) If this fails, then depending on the haemodynamic features try offloading either instead of, or in addition to, dopamine.

Chronic heart failure: long-term management

(1) Modify cardiovascular risk factor profile, e.g. cigarette smoking, obesity.

(2) Underlying causes should be treated, e.g. arrhythmias, hypertension.

(3) If this proves inadequate, or when there is no treatable underlying cause, diuretics should be the first stage. The type of diuretic and dose depends on severity of failure.

(4) If this proves inadequate, while some would still add digoxin, others nowadays would add an offloading agent either a nitrate, hydralazine or prazosin.

7.2 ANGINA PECTORIS

Aims

Relief of symptoms and particularly in unstable angina, prevention of progression to myocardial infarction.

Relevant pathophysiology

Angina is the symptom experienced when coronary blood supply is insufficient to meet myocardial energy requirements. Angina occurs in two forms:

(1) *Stable angina:* attacks are predictably provoked by exertion or excitement and recede when the increased energy demand is withdrawn. The underlying pathology is usually severe chronic coronary artery disease.

Treatment is undertaken on the assumption that the coronary obstructive disease is 'fixed'. Therefore, the opportunity for therapeutic benefit depends on adjustments in myocardial energy requirements and emphasis falls on drugs that reduce preload and afterload and which thus reduce metabolic demands.

(2) *Unstable angina:* attacks occur with lesser exertion or at rest and are unpredictable. The underlying pathology is often spasm or thrombus formation or extension in the coronary arteries.

Acute changes in coronary artery pathology are presumed and therapeutic attention directed to halting, reversing or bypassing the coronary arterial occlusive process in the hope of avoiding myocardial infarction. At the same time, treatment is aimed at reducing myocardial energy requirements.

Roughly one case in four of severe recent onset unstable angina progresses to myocardial infarction or death in the course of a few weeks. Although the outlook has improved with aggressive hospital management, not all cases respond. Where medical measures have evidently failed to stabilise or reverse the progress of severe unstable angina, coronary angiography and bypass surgery may be advisable on an urgent basis if infarction is to be prevented.

DRUGS USED IN ANGINA

Glyceryl trinitrate

Mechanism

A potent, direct, short-acting, smooth-muscle relaxant, with widespread vasodilator activity. In stable angina its major benefit results not from coronary artery dilatation, but probably depends on a brief drop in preload (venous return) by its action on venules and a reduced afterload by peripheral arteriolar relaxation.

In unstable angina, all these factors may be relevant but in addition, direct coronary artery dilation may also be important, particularly in those instances of variant rest angina in which coronary artery spasm can be demonstrated.

Pharmacokinetics

Virtually 100% first-pass metabolism and, it is, therefore, given sublingually. Very rapid clearance by liver metabolism: half-life about 2 min.

Adverse effects

These are dose related and result from vasodilation and reflex adverse effects to hypertension: headache, flushing and postural dizziness. These symptoms can be terminated by swallowing the tablet or spitting it out.

Clinical use and dose

Glyceryl trinitrate 0.5 mg tablets should be taken sublingually by the patient *before* carrying out a task known to produce angina. The total daily dose may be individually determined as that required to control symptoms. It may also be given transdermally in the form of a paste or ointment.

Isosorbide dinitrate

The clinical pharmacology is similar to glyceryl nitrate, but it is also effective orally and has a longer half-life of 40 min. It is used in the management of the acute phase of unstable angina.

Dose:

10 mg 8 hourly initially up to 30 mg 6 hourly. Maximum dose depends on symptomatic relief and adverse reactions of vaso-dilatation.

Beta-receptor blockers

The detailed clinical pharmacology of these drugs is described in Chapter 8.3.

Their value in angina depends mainly on decreasing myocardial oxygen consumption by:

(1) Limiting the increased heart rate associated with exercise, anxiety etc.,

(2) Limiting the increased force of contraction associated with the same stimuli.

In addition, beta-blockers can improve myocardial perfusion by their effect on heart rate, since tachycardia decreases the duration of diastole and, therefore, decreases the time available for effective coronary blood flow.

Adverse effects

These are described on p. 97. Rebound worsening of angina, myocardial infarction or serious tachydysrhythmias can occur if a beta-blocker is suddenly withdrawn from a patient in whom it was effectively controlling the angina. Always reduce the dose slowly in such patients.

Clinical use

Both stable and unstable angina. $Beta_1$-selective blocker drugs are currently preferred in unstable angina. This is because $beta_2$-receptors mediate vasodilation and if they are blocked then increased sympathetic activity results in unopposed vasoconstriction by an alpha-receptor effect.

Dose

See p. 99 for dose ranges of all beta-blockers.

Atenolol 50–200 mg daily	in an individually titrated dose to control symptoms and attenuate postural and exercise induced tachycardia.
Metoprolol 100–400 mg daily	
Propranolol 80–360 mg daily	

Calcium antagonists: nifedipine, verapamil.

Mechanism

Inhibition of the slow calcium-ion channel component of the muscle action potential leading to:

(1) Decreased contractility in myocardial cells, the main site of action of verapamil.

(2) Decreased tone in vascular smooth muscle cells including coronary arteries. The main effect of nifedipine.

(3) Verapamil has additional antiarrhythmic activity.

Pharmacokinetics

Both drugs are adequately absorbed following oral administration and are cleared by liver metabolism.

Adverse effects

Headache, nausea, flushing and postural dizziness.

Drug interactions

Verapamil should not be given with beta-blockers since the combined negative inotropic effects can precipitate heart failure.

Clinical use

Nifedipine is used both in stable and unstable angina. Dose is 10 mg, 8 hourly initially, increasing as required to control symptoms. Verapamil is of uncertain value in angina. Dose is 40 mg 8 hourly initially up to 120 mg 8 hourly.

GENERAL PRINCIPLES OF MANAGEMENT

Stable angina.
(1) Try to modify cardiovascular risk factors such as cigarette smoking, obesity.
(2) Treat any underlying precipitating cause such as anaemia, arrhythmias.
(3) Begin treatment with glyceryl trinitrate taken before undertaking the effort or activity which provokes pain.
(4) If unsuccessful, add a beta-blocker.
(5) If unsuccessful, use calcium antagonist either instead of or in addition to a beta-blocker.

Unstable angina: current aggressive regimes are under evaluation. Management typically involves combined treatment with a beta-blocker, isosorbide dinitrate and a calcium antagonist under close supervision in hospital. Patients not responding to this approach are submitted to early coronary arteriography and, if indicated, coronary artery surgery.

Comment

Angina pectoris is a subjective symptom of coronary artery disease. Where possible objective evidence of coronary disease should be sought using electrocardiography with or without exercise.

Treatment of angina is symptomatic with nitrates, beta-blockers and/or calcium antagonists. Any underlying cardiac or non-cardiac factors should be treated where possible.

CHAPTER 8

High blood pressure: hypertension

8.1   Relevant pathophysiology

8.2   Principles of drug treatment

8.3   Antihypertensive drugs

Aims

To reverse the hypertension-related increase in cardiovascular morbidity and mortality by long-term reduction of arterial pressure to an acceptable level which depends on age and sex, but is usually 140/90 mmHg or less.

8.1   RELEVANT PATHOPHYSIOLOGY

Blood pressure is the hydrostatic pressure within the systemic arteries and is determined by cardiac output and total peripheral resistance. There is no evidence of consistent increases in cardiac output or heart rate in hypertension. Total peripheral resistance is increased but the cause is not clear.

Blood pressure is normally or unimodally distributed in the population. There is no clear cut-off between normotensives and hypertensives. Long-term prospective studies indicate that for both systolic and diastolic blood pressure, the higher the pressure the greater the risk of cardiovascular disease. The frequency of hypertension depends on the arbitrary cut-off point selected, and varies with age, sex and social and environmental aspects of the population studied.

A practical definition of hypertension could be *that level of pressure at or above which long-term antihypertensive treatment is acknowledged to reduce cardiovascular morbidity.*

Hypertension is either *primary* or *secondary*. Even in younger age groups high blood pressure is *primary, idiopathic* or *essential* with no obvious cause in over 90% of patients. There is a strong polygenic familial trend with superimposed environmental and social factors.

Less commonly hypertension is *secondary* to renal or endocrine disease including:

(1) Acute or chronic renal disease (particularly glomerulo-nephritis),

(2) Renal artery stenosis (atheroma in older age group, fibromuscular hyperplasia in younger group),

(3) Hyperaldosteronism,

(4) Cushing's syndrome,

(5) Acromegaly,

(6) Phaeochromocytoma,

(7) Drugs:
> oral contraceptives,
> oestrogens,
> steroids,
> carbenoxolone,
> sympathomimetics

Risks of hypertension

Both *systolic* and *diastolic* blood pressure predict the likelihood of cardiovascular disease. Increased blood pressure is associated with increased morbidity and mortality from:

(1) Cerebrovascular disease, especially haemorrhagic strokes,

(2) Progressive chronic renal failure,

(3) Coronary artery disease: angina and myocardial infarction,

(4) Hypertensive congestive heart failure,

(5) Peripheral vascular disease.

There is a direct relationship between the severity of hypertension and the increase in morbidity. *Mild hypertension* carries an increased risk of these complications. *Moderately raised blood pressure* has a higher risk and *malignant hypertension* (severe hypertension with fibrinoid necrosis causing proteinuria and retinal haemorrhages, soft exudates or papilloedema) if untreated leads to death from cerebral haemorrhage or renal failure in over 90% of patients within 1 year.

Hypertension is an important risk factor but not the only cardiovascular risk predictor. Other identified risk factors include:

(1) Cigarette smoking,

(2) Obesity and glucose intolerance,

(3) Hyperlipidemia,

(4) Family history of vascular disease.

These factors have independent, additive effects on cardiovascular morbidity.

Benefits of treatment

The justification for treatment of hypertension by lowering blood pressure depends on the demonstration of improvements in cardio-vascular morbidity and mortality with long-term antihypertensive therapy.

(1) The benefits are well established in:

(a) Malignant or accelerated hypertension at any age,

(b) Severe hypertension (blood pressure > 200 mmHg systolic and/or 110 mmHg diastolic) at least in those under 65 years of age.

(2) There is now evidence of benefit in moderate hypertension (systolic 160–199 mmHg and/or diastolic 100–109 mmHg),

(3) The benefits of treatment are less well established and there remains controversy in:

(a) Mild hypertension (systolic 140–159 mmHg and/or diastolic 90–99 mmHg),

(b) Hypertension in the elderly.

Comment

The decision to treat mild–moderate hypertension is influenced by age and other risk factors: hypertension must be seen in the context of a person's overall cardiovascular risk profile.

8.2 PRINCIPLES OF DRUG TREATMENT

(1) Hypertension should be confirmed by several measurements of blood pressure.

(2) Hypertension should be treated as a part of a management plan for *all* identifiable risk factors.

(3) Non-pharmacological approaches should always be considered when appropriate:

(a) If obese, weight reduction of 10 kg lowers blood pressure 20/10 mmHg on average,

(b) If salt intake is very high (> 200 mEq/day) a modest reduction (by avoiding salty foods and table salt) may aid blood pressure control.

(4) The patient should be counselled about hypertension and its risks, and the case for long-term treatment should be carefully explained.

(5) A simple drug regimen, without unacceptable adverse effects or toxicity, should be established.

(6) Regular convenient long-term follow-up should be arranged *with blood pressure measurements.*

Stepped care programme

The simplest drug regimens are the most successful. Drugs should be given alone or in rational combinations which do not lead to adverse effects. Patient compliance is improved if drugs are only given once or twice daily. A widely used approach involves three steps:

Start treatment with one drug:

Step 1 Beta-blocker or thiazide diuretic

If monotherapy is unsuccessful then try both drugs:

Step 2 Beta-blocker *plus* thiazide diuretic

Step 1 or Step 2 controls blood pressure in 75–80% of patients.

For the remainder who are still not adequately controlled:

Step 3 Beta-Blocker *plus* thiazide diuretic *plus* vasodilator or alpha-blocker.

Triple therapy controls most of the remaining patients who take their tablets reliably (good compliers). Resistance to triple therapy is an indication for investigation of possible secondary renal or endocrine hypertension.

Resistant hypertension

Patients resistant to triple therapy may respond to the powerful vasodilator, minoxidil, with a beta blocker and loop diuretic, or alternatively to the converting enzyme inhibitor, captopril, with a diuretic.

Comment

The management of hypertension is a long-term undertaking, often in asymptomatic patients. The simplest, safest regimen should be determined for each individual.

Reduction of blood pressure and control of other risk fastors, like smoking and obesity, is undertaken to improve cardiovascular morbidity and mortality, without impairing the quality of life.

Emergency reduction of blood pressure

There are no indications for rapid, uncontrolled (within seconds or minutes) reduction of blood pressure. There remain a few indications for *controlled* moderate reduction (over minutes and hours). These include:

(1) Hypertensive encephalopathy,
(2) Eclampsia of pregnancy,
(3) Hypertensive acute left ventricular failure,
(4) Malignant or accelerated hypertension.

In many patients treatment can be given orally (beta-blocker and vasodilator), and blood pressure falls over the following 1–2 hours.

Intravenous drug administration although frequently used is only rarely necessary.

Sodium nitroprusside. This is given as a continuous titrated intravenous infusion. This has a short duration of action (1–2 min) so precipitous and prolonged falls in pressure, which may cause cerebrovascular accidents, can be avoided. The starting dose is 1 μg/kg/min and is increased until the desired effect is obtained. The infusion rate varies from 200–400 μg/min. Treatment for longer than 1–2 days may lead to accumulation of thiocyanate and poisoning, especially in patients with impaired renal function.

Diazoxide. This is a powerful vasodilator that should be given as multiple repeated intravenous doses of 50 or 100 mg as required and *not* as a single 300 mg dose, which often causes profound and uncontrolled hypotension.

Treatment of secondary hypertension

Medical treatment of secondary hypertension may be specifically tailored to the underlying abnormality of blood pressure control.

Chronic renal disease: as for essential hypertension but *caution* should be exercised over the dose of drugs that are usually excreted unchanged in urine, e.g. atenolol. Frusemide, not thiazides, should be used in severe renal failure.

Renovascular hypertension. This is a renin- (and angiotensin II) dependent hypertension. Converting enzyme inhibitors (captopril), which reduce angiotensin II formation or beta-blockers, which reduce renin release, are indicated. Consider surgical reconstruction.

Primary hyperaldosteronism (*Conn's Syndrome*). The competitive aldosterone antagonist spironolactone in large dose may be useful. Trilostane, an inhibitor of aldosterone biosynthesis, is under evaluation. Consider surgical removal of adenoma.

Phaeochromocytoma. Use alpha-receptor blockade with the non-competitive alpha-blocker phenoxybenzamine or the competitive alpha-blocker prazosin, together with a cardioselective beta-blocker (atenolol or metoprolol) if necessary for preoperative or intraoperative control of blood pressure and heart rate. *Never* give a beta-blocker alone: unopposed alpha-receptor stimulation can cause severe hypertension. In malignant phaeochromocytoma, which is inoperable, catecholamine synthesis may be reduced by alpha-methyl-paratyrosine.

8.3   ANTIHYPERTENSIVE DRUGS

Beta-adrenoceptor antagonists (beta-blockers)

Beta-blockers were developed as competitive antagonists of the effect of catecholamines on beta-receptors in the heart and other tissues. Their antihypertensive effect was noted in the early 1960s during clinical studies with propranolol in angina and cardiac arrhythmias. Early agents (propranolol and oxprenolol) blocked both

TABLE 8.1   Pharmacplogical properties, route of excretion and dose range of beta-blockers.

Approved name	Other actions			Major route of elimination	Daily dose (range in mg)
	Cardioselectivity	Intrinsic	Membrane activity		
Propranolol	−	−	+	Liver	40–320
Oxprenolol	−	+ +	+	Liver	40–320
Pindolol	−	+ +	+	Liver	10–30
Sotalol	−	−	−	Liver	200–480
Timolol	−	−	+	Liver	15–45
Nadolol	−	−	−	Kidney	80–240
Labetalol	−	−	+	Liver	300–2400
Atenolol	+ +	−	−	Kidney	50–200
Metoprolol	+ +	−	+	Liver	100–400
Acebutolol	+	+ +	+	Liver	400–1200

cardiac beta$_1$-receptors and beta$_2$-receptors in lung and peripheral vessels. More recent 'cardioselective' drugs (atenolol and metoprolol) have a *relatively* selective action on beta$_1$ receptors. There are now many beta-blockers available for clinical use with a range of selectivity and other properties (Table 8.1).

Mechanism

Beta-blockers antagonise the effects of noradrenaline and adrenaline on beta-receptors in a range of organs and tissues.

Heart. The responses to sympathetic nerve stimulation or circulating catecholamines are mediated by beta-receptors.

(1) Beta$_1$-receptors in the SA node have positive chronotropic actions. Blockade leads to bradycardia. Bradyarrhythmias are an adverse effect, especially in the elderly, because of decreased AV conduction.

(2) Beta$_1$-receptors in myocardium have a positive inotropic action. Blockade leads to an acute fall in cardiac output, not always maintained during chronic therapy, and a reduction in cardiac work, which may lead to precipitation or exacerbation of cardiac failure.

Acute haemodynamic effects of beta-blockers vary. Non-selective beta-blockers cause a substantial fall in cardiac output and a small fall in resting heart rate but a large fall in exercise heart rate. Peripheral resistance may be acutely increased. Chronic therapy may reduce cardiac output, but peripheral resistance and, therefore, blood pressure are lowered. Beta-blockers cause a fall in cardiac work and a reduction in myocardial oxygen demands, which justify their use in angina pectoris (Chapter 7.2).

Kidney. Beta-receptors control the release of renin from the juxtaglomerular cells of the kidney after renal nerve stimulation. Beta-blockers lower renin release and thus angiotensin II formation and aldosterone release.

Peripheral blood vessels. Beta$_2$-receptors in peripheral vessels subserve a vasodilator role especially in muscle beds. Blockade of beta$_2$-receptors may lead to cold hands and feet, Raynaud's phenomenon and worsening of peripheral vascular disease.

Bronchial smooth muscle. Beta$_2$-receptors cause dilatation of bronchial smooth muscle. Blockade may precipitate an acute attack of asthma in a susceptible person.

Central nervous system. Beta-receptors in the brain may be involved in blood pressure regulation and in other higher functions. Blockade of central beta-receptors may cause nightmares, vivid dreams and, rarely, hallucinations.

Other tissues. Uterus: stimulation of beta$_2$-receptors relaxes the gravid uterus and beta$_2$-agonists may be used to delay premature labour. *Eye:* beta$_2$-receptors control formation of aqueous humour.

In addition to blockade of beta-receptors these drugs may have other pharmacological effects (Table 8.1).

(1) Intrinsic sympathomimetic activity or partial agonist activity (oxprenolol, pindolol),

(2) Membrane-stabilising activity, quinidine-like or local anaesthetic effect (propranolol, oxprenolol),

(3) Alpha-receptor blockade (labetalol),

(4) Cardioselectivity or relatively greater blockade of beta$_1$-than beta$_2$-receptors (atenolol, metoprolol).

Cardioselectivity may reduce adverse effects resulting from beta$_2$-blockade. Membrane-stabilising activity is unlikely to contribute to the effects of beta-blockers in man. The relevance of intrinsic sympathomimetic activity is controversial. Co-existing alpha-blockade may be useful in more severe hypertension.

Pharmacokinetics

Beta-blockers are usually given orally except for rapid control of arrhythmias. As a group they show a wide variation in absorption, distribution, metabolism and elimination. The major determinants of these differences are:

(1) Hepatic metabolism, first-pass metabolism and systemic clearance,

(2) The role of the kidneys in elimination,

(3) Lipid solubility or ability to cross the blood–brain barrier.

Hepatic metabolism. Several beta-blockers show extensive first-pass metabolism after oral administration and uptake from the portal venous system (propranolol, oxprenolol, labetalol). These drugs are extensively metabolised by the liver. Propranolol is an example of a drug whose elimination depends on hepatic blood flow and is thus flow limited (p. 17). Wide differences in response between individuals are observed with variable bioavailability. There is a relatively wide range of doses required in clinical practice.

Renal elimination. Other beta-blockers (atenolol, nadolol) are eliminated almost entirely unchanged by the kidney. The dose range is relatively narrow, and it should be reduced and/or the frequency of administration adjusted in patients with renal impairment.

Lipid solubility. This determines the distribution of the drug across cell membranes in general, and across the blood–brain barrier in particular.

Propranolol and oxprenolol have a high lipid solubility, penetrate the brain and are present there in large amounts. They often cause nightmares, vivid dreams etc.

Atenolol and nadolol are both polar (non-lipid soluble) drugs. They cross the blood–brain barrier less readily and accumulate to a lesser extent in the nervous system.

Half-life. The half-life of most beta-blockers is short (< 4 h) but is longer for atenolol, nadolol and sotalol. The half-life, however, is only one factor contributing to duration of action, which depends on the magnitude and intensity of effect and thus also on the dose given. All beta-blockers given in a large enough dose act for 24 h, but drugs given in large dose because of their short half-life may cause adverse effects at early times corresponding to peak drug levels. Drugs like propranolol and metoprolol should be given twice daily. Long-acting or slow-release formulations are more expensive than standard formulations and have few objective advantages.

Adverse effects

These are often predictable and result from blockade of beta-receptors.

(1) Tiredness, fatigue and weakness,

(2) Bradycardia and heart block,

(3) Bronchospasm especially in asthmatics,

(4) Vivid dreams, nightmares and hallucinations,

(5) Congestive cardiac failure,

(6) Cold hands, Raynaud's phenomenon and worsening claudication,

(7) Loss of symptoms of hypoglycaemia in insulin dependent diabetics.

Beta-blockers may cause impotence in males by an unknown mechanism. There is *no indication* that the oculomucocutaneous syndrome which occurred in some patients treated with practolol is seen after any other beta-blockers.

Drug interactions

Hypertension as a result of unopposed peripheral alpha-adrenoceptor vasoconstriction.

(1) Beta-blockers may increase the severity of withdrawal hypertension if concurrent clonidine treatment is interrupted.

(2) Sympathomimetic amines amphetamine, ergotamine, ephedrine and phenylpropanolamine may cause severe hypertension reactions. The latter may be included in 'over the counter' proprietary cold cures.

Myocardial depression (prenylamine) or interference with conducting mechanisms (verapamil) causing asystole may complicate combined treatment with beta-blockers.

Cimetidine decreases hepatic metabolism of propranol and may increase effects like bradycardia. However, as the therapeutic range is wide, interactions involving metabolism or protein binding do not often lead to serious clinical consequences.

Clinical use and dose

Hypertension. Long-term treatment with all beta-blockers lowers blood pressure if an appropriate dose is given. Most beta-blockers can be given once or at the most twice daily with adequate blood pressure control. It is not clear whether the fall in blood pressure results from blockade of cardiac, renal or central nervous system beta-receptors.

Beta-blockers are widely used alone as first-line treatment in mild or moderate hypertension, or in combination with other drugs (thiazide diuretics, vasodilators, etc.) in more severe hypertension. The attenuation of the rise in heart rate after standing or exercise assists in selection of the dose and assessment of patient compliance.

Cardioselective drugs (atenolol, metoprolol) are useful if beta-blockers are used in the treatment of asthmatic or diabetic patients, or in those with peripheral vascular disease. Polar (non-lipid soluble) drugs such as atenolol are less likely to cause central adverse effects.

Atenolol: 50–200 mg once daily.
Metoprolol: 100–300 mg once or twice daily.
Propranolol: 40–320 mg once or twice daily.
Oxprenolol: 40–320 mg once or twice daily.

Comment

A simple once or twice daily regimen with beta-blockers encourages compliance in many patients and is effective and well tolerated. All beta-blockers lower blood pressure if given in an adequate dose. Cardioselective drugs are less likely to cause respiratory, metabolic and peripheral vascular adverse effects.

Arrhythmias (Chapter 6.3).

Angina pectoris (Chapter 7.2).

Anxiety neurosis (Chapter 18.1).

Thyrotoxicosis (Chapter 20.2).

Glaucoma. Beta-blockers may be used as eye drops (or systemically) in chronic simple glaucoma to reduce rate of formation of aqueous humour.

Diuretics

Mechanism

These agents increase urine volume and often sodium excretion by actions on salt and water transport across renal tubular and other cell membranes.

Several groups of diuretic drugs, with different sites of action, have been found to lower blood pressure (Table 8.2). Efficacy as an antihypertensive is not directly related to diuretic potency, and blood pressure lowering may result from a different action on vascular smooth muscle.

Thiazides are weak diuretics but useful antihypertensives. Diaxozide, a close structural analogue, actually causes sodium retention but is a powerful vasodilator antihypertensive. Frusemide and loop diuretics are potent diuretics with only modest effects on blood pressure.

Thiazides are the diuretic treatment of choice in uncomplicated hypertension with normal renal function. Loop diuretics and aldosterone antagonists have an important role in the treatment of the refractory oedema of heart failure (Chapter 7.1) and cirrhosis with ascites.

In hypertensive patients potent loop diuretics such as frusemide are only indicated:

(1) In chronic renal failure when thiazides are inactive,

(2) In hypertension resistant to standard triple therapy including a thiazide,

(3) In combination with vasodilators or captopril in severe resistant hypertension,

(4) In co-existing refractory congestive cardiac failure.

Potassium sparing diuretics have few advantages in uncomplicated hypertension. In patients with renal impairment they may cause hyperkalaemia and cardiac arrhythmias.

Pharmacokinetics

Thiazides are well absorbed orally, widely distributed, and subject to some hepatic metabolism. Renal actions depend on excretion of the drug into the tubule. Thus thiazides may be ineffective diuretics in severe renal impairment. The onset of diuretic action may be observed within 60 min and may last for 12 h or more. With

TABLE 8.2 Classification and mechanisms of actions of diuretics

	Mechanism	Comment
THIAZIDES Bendrofluazide Hydrochlorothiazide Chlorthalidone Clopamide Cyclopenthiazide Indapamide Polythiazide Zipamide	?Distal tubule ?Proximal tubule	All have an anti-hypertensive effect. Little evidence that newer agents have any advantages over older established agents.
LOOP DIURETICS Frusemide Bumetanide Ethacrynic acid	Ascending limb of loop of Henle	Potent diuretic and saluretic. Hypo-kalaemia frequent.
POTASSIUM SPARING DIURETICS Spironolactone Triampterene Amiloride	Aldosterone antagonist Distal tubule Sodium: potassium exchange	Useful in combination with thiazides or loop diuretics in refractory oedema. Also alone in hyperaldosteronism. May cause hyperkalaemia in renal failure or in the elderly.

repeated dosing the acute diuretic effect may be lost. The antihypertensive effect develops gradually over days, and it may take weeks or months to reach a maximum. The duration of antihypertensive effect is long (>24 h) permitting once daily dosing. The dose response curve is flat, and a simple regimen of one or two tablets achieves the maximum effect.

Adverse effects

Hypokalaemia. This may precipitate cardiac arrhythmias, especially in patients also on digoxin. Potassium supplements may be necessary (potassium chloride 1.2 g twice or more times daily) in these patients. Formulations that combine potassium with a diuretic seldom include a large enough supplemental dose. Severe hypokalaemia caused by thiazide suggests mineralocorticoid excess, i.e. a secondary cause for hypertension.

Hyperuricaemia. Inhibition of renal urate excretion raises serum uric acid and may provoke acute gouty arthritis.

Hyperglycaemia. Long-term diuretic therapy impairs glucose tolerance by inhibiting release of insulin from the pancreas. Normal glucose tolerance may become mildly diabetic and control is worsened in clinical diabetes.

Hypercalcaemia. This is a rare adverse effect resulting from reduced renal calcium excretion.

Impotence and reduced male sexual activity has recently been noted to be common with diuretics. The mechanism is not known.

Other adverse effects include skin rash, and thrombocytopenia.

Doses
Bendrofluazide: 5 or 10 mg twice daily.
Hydrochlorthiazide: 25–100 mg once daily.
Chlorthalidone: 25–100 mg once daily or on alternate days.

Comment

Thiazide diuretics alone or together with a beta-blocker are widely used, effective antihypertensives in mild, moderate and severe hypertension. Thiazides have a long duration of action favouring once daily dosing and a flat dose-response curve permitting simple standardised regimens. Routine potassium supplements are not usually required in uncomplicated hypertensives taking a normal diet with normal gastrointestinal function. Loop diuretics like frusemide with potassium supplements may be required in the management of resistant hypertension or chronic renal failure.

Vasodilators

Vasodilators appear to reverse a primary abnormality of hypertension (increased peripheral resistance). Their use alone in the long-term is limited by reflex compensatory mechanisms antagonising the fall in blood pressure and resulting in frequent, severe adverse effects. Reflex increases in sympathetic activity raise heart rate, cardiac output, renin and thus aldosterone release with sodium retention. These effects can be prevented by giving beta-blockers and diuretics with the vasodilator as triple therapy.

Drugs may act preferentially on arterioles (hydralazine) or veins (nitrates) or have a mixed effect (sodium nitroprusside). Vasodilators are also used in the treatment of heart failure and are considered in detail in Chapter 7.1.

Some act by identified mechanisms on specific receptors:

Alpha-receptor blockade: prazosin, labetalol.

Calcium slow-channel blockade: nifedipine, verapamil.

Others act 'non-specifically' by unknown mechanisms: hydralazine, minoxidil, diazoxide.

Hydralazine

Mechanism

This is a hydrazine derivative with a direct non-specific vasodilator action on arteriolar smooth muscle. It is widely used together with a beta-blocker and a diuretic in hypertension not responding to simpler regimens.

Pharmacokinetics

It is rapidly absorbed and distributed widely. The plasma half-life is short, but persistent binding of the drug to smooth muscle ensures a longer (>12 h) duration of effect. Hydralazine is metabolised by acetylation in the liver by the same genetically determined enzyme system as isoniazid, procainamide, dapsone, etc. Acetylator phenotype is an important determinant of response to drug (fast acetylators have a poor response), and also of toxicity (drug-induced lupus is rare in fast acetylators). Phenotyping may aid in determining safe upper limits of dosing: 200 mg in slow acetylators, 400 mg in fast acetylators.

Adverse effects

(1) Facial flushing and conjunctival injection: peripheral vasodilation.

(2) Weight gain and oedema from salt and water retention: a result of secondary hyperaldosteronism and direct effects on renal function.

(3) Headache: throbbing and *vascular* type (Chapter 19.3).

(4) Palpitations and tachycardia result from increased reflex drive and may aggravate angina or provoke myocardial infarction.

(5) Drug-induced lupus syndrome. Fever, arthralgia, malaise and hepatitis associated with positive antinuclear antibody test but normal DNA binding. The syndrome is similar to the connective tissue disease, systemic lupus erythematosis, but it is reversible and only rarely has renal or neurological features. It occurs mainly in slow acetylators with specific HLA tissue type and is uncommon if the dose is less than 200 mg daily.

Dose

Hydralazine: 25–100 mg twice daily, higher doses may be given in fast acetylators.

Calcium antagonists

These agents (nifedipine, verapamil) interfere with the action of interacellular calcium on both smooth and cardiac muscle. They are also used in the treatment of angina (see Chapter 7.2).

Recently the peripheral vasodilator effects of calcium antagonists have been utilised in the treatment of hypertension either alone or in combination therapy.

The common adverse effects of both agents, which result from reflex responses to peripheral vasodilation, can be countered by beta-blockers (flushing, headache) or diuretics (fluid retention). Verapamil may cause cardiac conduction abnormalities and congestive cardiac failure because of a direct cardiac depressant action.

Dose

Nifedipine: 10–40 mg twice or three times daily.
Verapamil: 40–120 mg twice or three times daily usually with beta-blocker or diuretic.

Minoxidil

A potent vasodilator which, used with beta-blockers and loop diuretics, is effective even in hypertension resistant to other drug combinations.

Severe fluid retention and oedema may require large (200–600 mg) doses of frusemide. Excess hair growth on face and limbs limits the acceptability of minoxidil in women.

Comment

Vasodilator drugs *given with* beta-blockers and diuretics are an effective and generally well-tolerated regimen for severe hypertension.

Alpha-receptor blockers

Prazosin

Mechanism

A competitive alpha-receptor blocker of the classical (alpha$_1$) vascular receptor at the doses and plasma levels observed clinically. Prazosin acts on both arteriolar and venous resistance, and may cause less reflex cardiac stimulation and renin release than hydralazine.

While prazosin could be used alone in mild hypertension, it is more often employed in combination with beta-blockers or diuretics. It is always started cautiously with low doses because of orthostatic hypotension and syncope, which may be severe after the first dose.

Pharmacokinetics

Prazosin is well absorbed orally and subject to first-pass extraction and liver metabolism. The half-life is short (2–3 h) but longer duration of action permits twice daily dosing.

Adverse effects

Postural hypotension with syncope may occur after the first dose of prazosin or with dose increments. Postural effects usually wear off but occasionally may persist in the elderly, or at high doses with both prazosin and labetalol. Drowsiness and weakness may rarely occur.

Dose

Prazosin: 0.5 mg before bedtime as the first dose then 1–10 mg twice daily by individual titration of dose as required to control blood pressure.
Labetalol: 100 mg twice or three times daily increasing as required to 2.4 g daily in divided doses.

Centrally-acting drugs

Methyldopa (via an active metabolite, methylnoradrenaline) and clonidine (directly) act on $alpha_2$-receptors in the brain stem to reduce efferent sympathetic tone and blood pressure.

Adverse effects

Both clonidine and methyldopa have other CNS effects including drowsiness, sedation and depression resulting from actions on other central $alpha_2$-receptors. They also cause dry mouth. Interference with sexual activity and impotence in men is not uncommon.

Postural hypotension may occur with methyldopa, especially in the elderly. It causes a positive direct antiglobulin test and rarely haemolytic anaemia. Drug-induced hepatitis with fever may occur within the first few weeks of methyldopa treatment or on rechallenge.

If clonidine treatment is interrupted or stopped suddenly a hypertensive reaction with sweating, anxiety, tremor etc. may occur within 24–36 h.

Dose

Methyldopa: 250–1000 mg twice daily.
Clonidine: 100–600 μg twice daily.

Comment

Centrally-acting drugs are being less widely used now as there are alternative agents of comparable efficacy with fewer adverse effects. Methyldopa may be used as an alternative to beta-blockers or diuretics where the first choice drug is contraindicated or poorly tolerated.

Converting enzyme inhibitors

Mechanism

Captopril has been recently introduced for severe or resistant hypertension. It acts by competitively blocking angiotensin converting enzyme (kininase II) and preventing the formation of angiotensin II. Captopril is particularly effective when plasma renin activity (and thus angiotensin II) is raised as in renovascular hypertension. In resistant hypertension captopril, together with a diuretic, may be successful. In sodium depleted patients captopril should be started at very low doses as severe hypotension may occur.

Adverse effects

Limited experience indicates that skin rash and loss of taste occur in about 10% of patients.

More serious adverse effects: leucopenia and proteinuria, have been observed in a small number of patients.

Dose

Captopril: 25–75 mg twice or three times daily with or without diuretic (thiazide or frusemide). Lower doses may be indicated in renal failure.

Comment

Captopril may be useful in resistant hypertension or renovascular hypertension and is often given with a diuretic. Until the incidence of serious adverse effects is clear, it is not suitable for widespread use in mild to moderate hypertension.

Antimicrobial therapy

Aim

Eradication of organisms without damage to the patient.

One of the greatest of all therapeutic advances was the introduction of drugs that eradicated bacterial infections in man. The introduction of sulphonamides in 1936 and penicillins in 1941 dramatically reduced mortality from infections. During the decades since then there has been a vast increase in the number of antimicrobials available for clinical use. This ready availability of drugs has enhanced the likelihood that a suitable agent can be found for a particular infection, but it has also resulted in a confusing range of choice and a readiness to prescribe antimicrobials even when the presence of bacterial infection is poorly documented.

TABLE 9.1   General principles of antimicrobial therapy

Patient	Organism	Drug
Document infection	Culture	Absorption
Factors altering kinetics:	Identification	Tissue distribution
age; renal/hepatic function	Typing	Route of elimination
Previous drug sensitivity	Sensitivity	Adverse reactions
General health (resistance		Drug interactions
to infection)		
Pregnancy		

9.1 PRINCIPLES OF DRUG TREATMENT

The patient

Documentation of infection

Whenever possible the clinical suspicion of infection should be supported by laboratory diagnosis. Relevant samples, e.g. sputum, urine or blood, should be obtained before treatment is commenced.

Age

Drug kinetics are influenced by age dependent changes in pathways of elimination (Chapter 3). Clinically important examples involving antimicrobials include:

(1) Relative deficiency of hepatic glucuronyl transferase in neonates leading to accumulation of chloramphenicol with likelihood of cardiovascular collapse.

(2) Physiological decrease in renal function with age leading to accumulation of aminoglycosides in the elderly with likelihood of toxicity: dose modification is necessary.

Other antimicrobials contraindicated in specific age groups are:

(3) Sulphonamides in the neonate (displacement of bilirubin leading to kernicterus).

(4) Tetracyclines in growing children (tooth discolouration).

Renal and hepatic function (Chapter 2.2)

Many commonly used antimicrobials are eliminated by the kidney while a few undergo hepatic metabolism. Dose modification is likely to be necessary if renal function is moderately or severely impaired (Table 9.2). Drug level monitoring is mandatory for antimicrobials with concentration related toxicity.

Drug sensitivity

Always ask about previous exposure to drugs. Penicillins and cephalosporins are the antimicrobials most frequently associated with sensitivity reactions and there is a 5–10% cross-sensitivity between these two drug groups. Sulphonamides also frequently cause allergic reactions.

Diminished resistance to infection

Patients with malignant disease or who are receiving cytotoxic or immunosuppressant drugs are susceptible to severe infections often with less common organisms, e.g. yeasts, fungi and protozoa. In particular, granulocytopaenia of less than $500 \times 10^6/l$ is accompanied by a high risk of septicaemia. Fever in such patients must be assumed to have an infective aetiology and should be treated aggressively before definitive bacteriological information is available.

Pregnancy (Chapter 4.1)

Penicillins and cephalosporins are not harmful to the fetus. Fetal damage has been definitely associated with streptomycin and the tetracyclines. Possible adverse fetal effects have been ascribed to gentamicin, kanamycin and co-trimoxazole.

Comment

The patient's age, sex and general state of health must be considered when choosing both the drug and its dose.

TABLE 9.2 (a) Antimicrobials for which dose modification is required in mild, moderate or severe renal failure

Mild	Moderate	Severe
Aminoglycosides (monitor levels)	Metronidazole	Co-trimoxazole
Amphotericin B	Carbenicillin	Penicillins
Cephalosporins (more recent)		
Ethambutol		*Avoid*: Cephalothin, cephaloridine,
Flucytosine		nalidixic acid, nitrofurantoin,
Vancomycin		talampicillin, tetracyclines

(b) Antimicrobials for which dose modification is required in liver disease

Clindamycin
Isoniazid
Rifampicin

Avoid: Erythromycin estolate,
pyrazinamide, talampicillin

The organism

Bacteria

Sensitivity. Bactericidal drugs destroy the organisms against which they are effective. Bacteriostatic drugs do not kill the organism but destroy ability to replicate. Use of a bacteriostatic drug assumes that body defences can destroy the organisms whose replication has been prevented. In-vitro testing is available for most antibacterial drugs. Application of in-vitro findings to the patient assumes that adequate drug concentrations are achieved at the site of infection.

Resistance. Some bacteria have always been resistant to the effects of certain drugs, while others have developed resistance in the course of repeated exposure to antimicrobials. The two major mechanisms by which resistance is produced are gene mutation and exchange of DNA between bacteria. Resistance may take the form of an alteration in the bacterial component on which the drug acts, e.g. changes in the 30S ribosomal subunit in organisms developing resistance to aminoglycosides. Alternatively the drug might be destroyed by the organisms, as in the case of penicillins which are inactivated by beta-lactamases produced by resistant bacteria.

The development of resistance can be reduced if antimicrobials are not given indiscriminately. Additionally, the use of drug combinations should limit the appearance of resistant organisms in conditions such as tuberculosis where prolonged treatment is necessary.

Viruses and fungi

The range of effective drugs is limited and in many cases treatment is still experimental. Consequently, information about sensitivity or resistance to treatment is far less complete than for bacteria. Organisms are considered individually under specific agents.

Comment

Antimicrobial treatment must take account of the organism's susceptibility to drugs *and* the patient's intrinsic ability to combat infection.

The drug

Absorption

Certain antimicrobials, for example the aminoglycosides, can only be given parenterally because absorption from the gastrointestinal tract is negligible. Where a choice exists between oral and parenteral drug formulations, the decision must rest on the severity of the illness and the need to achieve high tissue concentrations.

Tissue distribution

The principles determining drug distribution are described in Chapter 1.3. In addition to these general considerations of blood concentration, protein binding, lipid solubility etc., a further factor influencing antimicrobial distribution is the presence of inflammation which tends to improve tissue penetration. However, it must not be assumed that the presence of inflammation greatly transforms the penetration of drugs. For example, gentamicin and cephalosporins cross poorly into the CSF even in the presence of meningitis. Table 9.3 indicates those agents with high penetration of CSF, bile, urine and bone.

Route of elimination

This is renal, hepatic metabolism or (rarely) biliary excretion. See Chapter 2 and Section 9.1c above.

TABLE 9.3   Antimicrobials for which high concentrations are achieved

CSF	Bile	Urine
Chloramphenicol	Penicillins	Penicillins
Erythromycin	Cephalosporins	Cephalosporins
Isoniazid	Erythromycin	Aminoglycosides
Pyrazinamide		Sulphonamides
Rifampicin		Nitrofurantoin
5-fluorocytosine		Nalidixic acid
		Ethambutol
		5-fluorocytosine

Adverse effects

These are of two general types. Hypersensitivity reactions which are either immediate (lgE mediated) or delayed (lgG mediated). The former produce anaphylaxis, while the latter manifest themselves in various ways, the most common being rashes. Hypersensitivity reactions usually occur with no prior warning and are most commonly seen with penicillins, cephalosporins and sulphonamides.

The other type of adverse reaction is usually predictable in being concentration related; aminoglycoside ototoxicity is an example. Fortunately, the toxic concentrations of most antimicrobials in common use greatly exceed the required therapeutic concentrations. Where this is not the case, e.g. gentamicin, drug level monitoring is mandatory. Adverse reactions to antimicrobials are summarised in Table 9.4 and discussed in more detail under specific agents.

Drug interactions

These can be either kinetic, e.g. enzyme induction or inhibition, or dynamic, e.g. two drugs adversely affecting the same organ.

Examples include:
(1) Aminoglycosides and frusemide have an additive nephrotoxic effect.
(2) Rifampicin induces the same enzymes that metabolise the contraceptive pill and can cause failure of contraception.
(3) Sulphonamides can inhibit the enzymes that metabolise phenytoin and can cause phenytoin toxicity.
(4) Tetracyclines form insoluble complexes in gut lumen with both antacids and iron leading to treatment failure.

Antimicrobial prophylaxis

Antimicrobials are sometimes given to people who do not have an infection but who are considered to be at risk from a specific organism. Examples include the use of minocycline or rifampicin in close contacts of patients with meningococcal meningitis, the administration of penicillin before and following dental procedures

TABLE 9.4   Major adverse reactions of antimicrobial drugs

Organ system	Drug	Comment
Kidney	Aminoglycosides	Concentration related
	Cephalosporins	Mainly earlier drugs of this group
	Sulphonamides	
	Methicillin	Other penicillins rarely
	Amphotericin B	
	Polymyxins	Limits use
Bone marrow suppression	Antiviral agents	
	Amphotericin B	
	Flucytosine	
	Chloramphenicol	
	Sulphonamides	Rare
Haemolytic anaemia	Sulphonamides	
	Nitrofurantoin	Two distinct mechanisms: immune and G-6-PD deficiency
	Nalidixic Acid	
	Penicillins	Rare
	Cephalosporins	Rare

Thrombocytopaenia	Sulphonamides	Rare
	Cephalosporins	Rare
Neutropaenia	Rifampicin	Intermittent therapy
	Penicillins	Rare: mainly ampicillin, carbenicillin
	Cephalosporins	Rare
	Sulphonamides Chloramphenicol	Rare
Neurological		
Eighth nerve	Aminoglycosides	Concentration related
	Vancomycin	
Optic nerve	Ethambutol	
Peripheral neuropathy	Isoniazid	Prevented by pyridoxine
	Metronidazole	Prolonged treatment
	Nitrofurantoin	
Convulsions	Penicillins	Large intrathecal or massive i.v. doses
	Cephalosporins	Large intrathecal doses
	Nalidixic acid	Large doses
Benign intracranial hypertension	Tetracyclines	
	Penicillins	
	Nalidixic acid	
Neuromusclar blockade	Aminoglycosides	

TABLE 9.4 (continued)

Organ system	Drug	Comment
Gastrointestinal System		
Liver	Isoniazid	More often rapid acetylators
	Rifampicin	Usually mild—worse in alcoholics/preceding damage
	Tetracyclines	Massive doses
	Erythromycin estolate	
	Nitrofurantoin	
	Penicillins	
Transient rise in transaminases	Cephalosporins	
Diarrhoea	Penicillins	Specially ampicillin
	Tetracyclines	
	Clindamycin	Pseudomembranous colitis (Cl. difficile).
Other adverse reactions		
Hypersensitivity	Penicillins	
	Cephalosporins	10% cross-sensitivity
	Sulphonamides	
Stevens–Johnson syndrome	Sulphonamides	
	Penicillins	
Bone development/tooth staining	Tetracyclines	Contraindicated in childhood
Pulmonary fibrosis	Nitrofurantoin	
Rashes	Commonly penicillins and sulphonamides but virtually any drug can cause rashes	

in people at risk of endocarditis, and the long-term use of co-trimoxazole in children with repeated urinary tract infections and evidence of vesicoureteric reflux.

Comment

An antimicrobial might be quite ineffective, or even dangerous, unless its clinical pharmacology is viewed in relation to the whole clinical situation. The drug chosen must reach the site of infection, in an effective concentration, without producing toxicity or adversely influencing any concurrent therapy.

9.2 ANTIBACTERIAL DRUGS (Table 9.5)

Penicillins

Mechanism

Penicillins have a bactericidal action. They inhibit cell wall synthesis by preventing formation of peptidoglycan cross bridges.

Pharmacokinetics

Oral absorption. Not absorbed: carbenicillin, ticarcillin, mecillinam.

Moderately absorbed: benzylpenicillin (penicillin G), ampicillin, talampicillin, cloxacillin.

Well absorbed: phenoxypenicillin, amoxycillin, flucloxicillin, pivmecillinam.

Even relatively well absorbed penicillins are destroyed to some extent by gastric acid and should, therefore, be given at least 30 min before meals.

Distribution. The penicillins have good penetration to most tissues but poor entry to CSF. This is compensated for in treating meningitis by giving large doses intravenously.

Elimination. Undergoes enterohepatic circulation: drug is excreted via bile and reabsorbed. The major route of elimination after

TABLE 9.5 First and second line antibacterial drugs

Drug	Strep. Pneumoniae + Strep. pyoyenes	Strep. faecalis	Staph. aureus (Pen sensitive)	Staph. aureus (Pen resistant)	N. meningitis	N. gonorrheoae	H. influenzae	Salmonella typhi	Klebsiella pneumoniae	E. Coli	Proteus mirabilis	Pseudomonas	Bacteroides fragilis	Mycoplasma	Rickettsia	Legionella pneumophila	Chlamydia	Brucella
Penicillins	1		1		1	1[R]												
Ampicillin/Amoxycillin	1[a]	1	1				1[R]	1/2		1[R]	1							
Cloxacillin/Flucloxacillin	1		2	1														
Carbenicillin/Ticarcillin												2[R]						
Mecillinam																		
Cefuroxime/Cefotaxime	2	1[b]	2	2		2	1/2		1/2	2	2							
Co-trimoxazole	2		2[R]				2	2	2	1[b]	1						2	2
Erythromycin	2[R]		2[R]	2[R]			2							1/2		1	1	
Tetracyclines							2[R]							1/2	1	1	1	1
Gentamicin									1/2	1	1	1						
Metrinidazole													1[c]					
Chloramphenicol					2		1[d]	2	1		1		1/2		1			1

1 First line: where more than one drug is shown, the choice depends on disease severity and site.

2 Second line: either less effective or similar efficacy to first-line drug but more toxic or more expensive.

a Preferred when these organisms cause otitis media.

b Used against these bacteria mainly in localised infections, e.g. urinary tract or gall bladder.

c Effective against many other anaerobes.

d When this bacterium is causing meningitis.

R Resistant strains developing.

reabsorption is active secretion in the renal tubules. This tubular secretion can be blocked by probenecid with doubling of penicillin blood levels. Dose modification is necessary in severe renal failure.

Adverse effects

Immediate hypersensitivity. This occurs in 0.05% of patients with manifestations ranging from urticaria or wheezing to a life-threatening anaphylactic response.

Delayed hypersensitivity: This occurs in <5% of patients, mainly as rashes. Rare manifestations are haemolytic anaemia, leukopaenia, interstitial nephritis (mainly reported with methicillin). Cross-sensitivity with cephalosporins occurs in around 10% of patients.

Toxicity. Convulsions following large (> 15 000 units) intrathecal or very high (100 million units/day) intravenous doses of penicillin. Patients with renal insufficiency can develop cation overload following large doses of potassium penicillin or sodium carbenicillin. Diarrhoea is commonly reported, particularly with ampicillin (20%).

Note. Ampicillin has a unique adverse effect comprising a rash in up to 90% of patients with mononucleosis or chronic lymphatic leukaemia.

Drug interactions

Penicillins are largely free of important drug interactions. Only major exception is that ampicillin can lead to oral contraceptive failure probably because of diminished enterohepatic circulation.

Antibacterial spectrum

The major factor limiting efficacy is the production by certain organisms of enzymes (penicillinases) which destroy the beta-lactam ring of the penicillin molecule. This structure is essential to the antibacterial action of penicillins. Several synthetic penicillins incorporate side chains which protect the beta-lactam ring against these enzymes. However, this also has the effect of protecting bacteria from the beta-lactam ring. Penicillinase resistant drugs, therefore, are generally less effective than their penicillinase sensitive counterparts and are indicated only for the treatment of infection caused by penicillinase-producing staphylococci.

Penicillinase-sensitive penicillins. Benzylpenicillin and phenoxypenicillins are active against streptococci, *Neisseria, Treponema pallidum, Actinomyces israelii* and several anaerobic organisms but not *Bacteroides fragilis.* Ampicillin, amoxycillin and talampicillin have a broader spectrum and are effective against *E. coli, Shigella, Salmonella, Haemophilus influenzae, Proteus mirabilis* and various enterococci. Amoxycillin is somewhat better absorbed than ampicillin, but in practical terms there is little to choose between these three drugs. Their main indications are urinary tract infection, cholecystitis, acute exacerbations of chronic bronchitis and, parenterally (ampicillin) in *H. influenzae* meningitis (depending on sensitivity of organism).

Carbenicillin and ticarcillin are active against *Pseudomonas aeruginosa* and *Proteus* species. At least in-vitro ticarcillin is more effective than carbenicillin against *P. aeruginosa.* Both drugs must be given parenterally but the phenyl ester of carbenicillin (carfecillin) is effective orally. Bacterial resistance encountered in some strains. Mecillinam and its orally active ester pivmecillinam are effective against *Salmonella* species.

Penicillinase-resistant penicillins. Cloxacillin, flucloxacillin and methicillin are indicated only in the treatment of infections caused by penicillinase-producing staphylococci. Flucloxacillin is better absorbed from the gut than cloxacillin. More cases of interstitial nephritis have been reported following methicillin therapy than with any other penicillin.

Doses

Benzylpenicillin: intramuscular 300–600 mg 2–4 times daily (children 10–20 mg/kg daily). Intravenous up to 24 g daily. Intrathecal 6–12 mg daily.
Phenoxymethylpenicillin: oral dose 250–500 mg 6 hourly (children 125–250 mg 6 hourly).

Ampicillin: oral dose 250–1000 mg 6 hourly. Intravenous or intramuscular 500 mg–1000 mg 6 hourly (children half doses).
Amoxycillin: oral 250–500 mg 8 hourly (children half dose).
Talampicillin: oral 250–500 mg 8 hourly.
Carbenicillin: intravenous (rapid infusion) 5g 4–6 hourly (children 250–400 mg/kg daily divided doses). Intramuscular 2 g 6 hourly (children 50–100 mg/kg divided doses).
Ticarcillin: intravenous infusion (rapid) or intramuscular 15–20 g daily divided doses.
Mecillinam: slow intravenous injection or intramuscular 5–15 mg/kg 6 hourly.
Pivmecillinam: oral 1.2–2.4 g daily in salmonellosis.
Cloxacillin: intramuscular 500 mg 6 hourly, intravenous 500–1000 mg 6 hourly (children quarter to half dose).
Flucloxacillin: oral 250 mg 6 hourly.

Cephalosporins

Mechanism

Cephalosporins are bactericidal. They contain a beta-lactam ring and their mechanism of action is similar to penicillins.

Pharmacokinetics

Only three cephalosporins are effective orally: cephalexin, cephradine and cefaclor. They distribute widely but, except cephaloridine, not into the CSF, even in the presence of meningitis. The drugs are eliminated renally, partly by glomerular filtration and partly by tubular secretion, with the contribution of each route varying with individual cephalosporins.

Adverse effects

Hypersensitivity is the main adverse effect with around a 10% cross-reactivity with penicillin sensitive patients. Cephaloridine can cause renal tubular necrosis, particularly when given in doses above 6 g/day. A positive Coombs' test occurs in about 5% of patients receiving cephalothin but haemolytic anaemia is rare.

Drug interactions

The nephrotoxicity of cephaloridine is potentiated by loop diuretics and aminoglycoside antibiotics.

Antibacterial spectrum

Cephaloridine, cephalothin, cephazolin and the orally active cephalosporins are broad spectrum but with limited activity against Gram-negative organisms because of degradation by beta-lactamases produced by them (but not those produced by staphylococci). Cephamandole, cefuroxime and cefotaxime are more resistant to beta-lactamases and are effective against *H. influenzae,* with cefuroxime also being active against *N. gonorrhoeae.* Cefoxitin is closely related to the basic cephalosporin structure but is active against Gram-negative and anaerobic bacteria.

Doses

Oral: **Cephalexin and cephradine:** 250–500 mg 6 hourly (children 25–50 mg/kg/day in divided doses).

Intravenous: **Cephradine:** 500–1000 mg 6 hourly (children 50–100 mg/kg daily in 6 hourly doses).

Cephazolin: 500–1000 mg 6 hourly (children 125–250 mg 8 hourly).

Cefuroxime: 1.5 g 6 hourly (children 30–100 mg/kg daily in divided doses).

Cephamandole: 500–2000 mg 6 hourly (children 50–100 mg/kg daily in divided doses).

Cefotaxime: 1 g 12 hourly to 3 g 6 hourly depending on severity (children 100–200 mg/kg/day in divided doses).

Cefoxitin: 1–2 g 8 hourly (children 80–160 mg/kg daily in divided doses).

Comment

The cephalosporins are used extensively but in most infections for which a cephalosporin might be considered, another antibiotic is usually at least as effective, at least as safe and almost certainly much less expensive. Exceptions include certain infections caused by *Klebsiella pneumoniae* and *Staph. albus.*

Aminoglycosides

Mechanism

Aminoglycosides are bactericidal. They bind to 30S subunit of bacterial ribosomes leading to misreading of m-RNA codons.

Pharmacokinetics

Oral absorption is negligible. They have poor penetration into CSF and only moderate penetration to bile. Otherwise there is good entry to inflamed tissue. Elimination is mainly by glomerular filtration.

Adverse effects

There are two major adverse reactions, both concentration related: nephrotoxicity and ototoxicity. The renal lesion consists of tubular destruction. Eighth nerve damage can be mainly vestibular (streptomycin, gentamicin) or mainly auditory (kanamycin).

The severity of these reactions is related to aminoglycoside serum concentration which in turn is related to dose and rate of elimination. Accumulation of drug occurs when glomerular filtration is decreased by renal disease or at the extremes of age. Doses must be modified in these situations and drug concentration monitoring is mandatory. Aminoglycosides cross the placenta and can cause eighth nerve damage in the fetus. An uncommon effect of aminoglycosides is neuromuscular blockade occurring after rapid intravenous injection; this is most marked in patients with myasthaenia gravis (Chapter 19.4).

Drug interactions

Nephrotoxicity is enhanced by co-administration with cephaloridine or polymyxins. Similarly, ototoxicity is enhanced by loop diuretics. The neuromuscular blockade of curare-like drugs can be prolonged by aminoglycosides.

Antibacterial spectrum

Gentamicin is the major aminoglycoside and is active against all aerobic Gram-negative rods including *Pseudomonas* and *Proteus* and also against staphylococci. Most streptococci are resistant because gentamicin cannot penetrate the cell. However, penicillin and gentamicin have a synergistic effect against some streptococci. Anaerobic organisms are all resistant. Tobramycin is 2–4 times more active against Pseudomonas but is otherwise very similar to gentamicin. Amikacin is resistant to most of the bacterial enzymes which inactivate gentamicin and is only indicated for infections caused by aerobic Gram-negative rods against which gentamicin is no longer effective.

Neomycin is given orally to decrease the bacterial content of the colon in liver failure or prior to bowel surgery. If there is severe liver or renal failure or inflammatory bowel disease, sufficient neomycin can be absorbed to cause ototoxicity.

Streptomycin is effective against tubercle bacilli and is discussed later in the chapter.

Dose

Gentamicin: if renal function is normal, the intramuscular dose is 2–5 mg/kg daily given at 8 hourly intervals. Various nomograms and formulae are widely available for calculating dose modifications in renal impairment. A rough guide, based on creatinine clearance is:

Cr. Cl. (ml/min)	Dose interval (h)
> 70	8
30–70	12
10–30	24
5–10	48

It must be emphasised that rules of thumb are not a substitute for drug level monitoring.

Tobramycin: 3–5 mg/kg daily given in divided doses 8 hourly. Modify dose in renal failure.

Amikacin: 15 mg/kg daily in 12 hourly doses. Modify dose in renal failure.

Comment

The major role of aminoglycosides is the parenteral treatment of serious infection caused by sensitive organisms. These drugs are popular for the initial management of life threatening septicaemia of uncertain aetiology. In this situation an aminoglycoside is usually combined with metronidazole or carbenicillin.

Co-trimoxazole

Mechanism

These drugs are bactericidal. Co-trimoxazole contains a culphonamide, sulphamethoxazole, and trimethoprim in the ratio 5 : 1. The basis of the action of sulphonamides is that bacterial cells are impermeable to folic acid so must synthesise their own from para-aminobenzoic acid with which sulphonamides have a strong similarity. Thus competitive inhibition of folic acid synthesis occurs. Trimethoprim blocks the next synthetic step, from folic acid to tetrahydrofolate, by inhibiting the enzyme dihydrofolate reductase.

Pharmacokinetics

Co-trimoxazole is well absorbed following oral administration and is also available for intravenous use. There is wide tissue distribution and elimination is by renal excretion.

Adverse effects

The sulphonamide component can cause rashes and, much less commonly, Stevens–Johnson syndrome, renal failure and blood dyscrasias. Trimethoprim can also cause rashes and impaired haemopoiesis and can produce gastrointestinal symptoms. The trimethoprim component has been implicated in teratogenesis (cleft palate). In the newborn sulphonamides can displace bilirubin from protein-binding sites and cause kernicterus.

Drug interactions

The sulphonamide component competes for hepatic enzyme binding sites and can decrease the clearance of phenytoin, tolbutamide and warfarin sufficiently to produce phenytoin toxicity, hypoglycaemia and enhanced anticoagulation respectively. Displacement of methotrexate from protein binding sites can also lead to toxicity.

Antibacterial spectrum

Broad spectrum including Gram-positive cocci, *N. gonorrheoae*, *H. influenzae*, *E. coli*, *Proteus mirabilis*, *Shigella*, *Salmonella*, *Pneumocystis carinii* and *Brucella*.

Dose

Sulphamethoxazole 400 mg, **trimethoprim** 80 mg per tablet, two tablets 12 hourly in adults (children 120–480 mg 12 hourly depending on age).

Comment

Although broad in antibacterial spectrum, co-trimoxazole is currently the drug of first choice only in urinary tract infections caused by susceptible coliforms. However, it is a useful second-line drug in several situations where the usual agent is contraindicated because of adverse reactions or bacterial resistance. Examples include typhoid fever, exacerbations of chronic bronchitis and gonorrhoea in penicillin-sensitive patients.

Tetracyclines

Mechanism

Tetracyclines are bacteriostatic. Binding to 30S ribosomal subunit with consequent misreading of information for protein synthesis.

Pharmacokinetics

Adequately absorbed following oral administration. Tissue distribution is good and the drugs are eliminated mainly unmetabolised by biliary excretion.

Adverse effects

Tetracyclines bind to calcium in bones and teeth leading to impaired bone growth and discolouration of teeth during active mineralisation (up to 7 years). Tetracyclines cross the placenta and are contraindicated in pregnancy. Following large doses both hepatic necrosis and renal failure have been reported. Impairment of protein synthesis can lead to enhanced effects of catabolism in severe renal failure. Tetracyclines are contraindicated in renal failure. Many patients develop diarrhoea on tetracycline therapy.

Drug interactions

Both antacids and iron form insoluble complexes with tetracyclines in the gut lumen leading to treatment failure.

Antibacterial spectrum

The tetracyclines are effective against a wide range of bacteria but resistance is increasing, and they should no longer be considered useful broad spectrum antibiotics. The importance of tetracyclines is based on their efficacy against chlamydia (e.g. psittacosis), rickettsia (e.g. Q fever, typhus Rocky Mountain spotted fever), mycoplasma, brucella and cholera. In these infections tetracyclines are the drugs of first choice. Tetracyclines are also useful adjuncts to the treatment of acne by preventing growth of *Propionibacterium* acnes in the pustules. The other specific indication for a tetracycline is the use of minocycline for meningococcal prophylaxis.

Dose

Tetracycline and **oxytetracycline** 250–500 mg 6 hourly.
Minocycline: 200 mg then 100 mg 12 hourly.

Other antibacterial drugs

Metronidazole

Initially used in protozoal infections, especially *Trichomonas*, but also very effective against anaerobic bacteria, particularly *Bacteroides fragilis*. It is currently popular in treating serious anaerobic infections. In addition, metronidazole is often combined with gentamicin in treating serious mixed infections or septicaemia of uncertain aetiology. The other major uses are in treating trichomonal vaginitis, amoebiasis and giardiasis. Only major adverse effects are peripheral neuropathy following prolonged therapy and seizures following high doses.

Dose

For severe infections, intravenous infusion at the rate of 500 mg every 8 hours in adults and 7.5 mg/kg 12 hourly in children for 7 days. Oral: 200 mg 8 hourly for 7 days for trichomoniasis and 2 g daily for 3 days in amoebiasis and giardiasis. If appropriate, suppositories can be used in circumstances where i.v. infusion might be considered: similar blood levels but much cheaper. Dose: 1 g 8 hourly.

Erythromycin

Antibacterial spectrum similar to penicillin and is a suitable second-line drug for patients allergic to penicillin. Erythromycin is currently drug of choice for *Legionella pneumophilia*. It is of some value on whooping cough prophylaxis and is effective against *Mycoplasma*. Only major adverse effect is cholestatic jaundice associated with the estolate formulation. This formulation is therefore contraindicated in liver disease.

Dose

Oral: 250–500 mg 6 hourly for adults, 125–250 mg 6 hourly for children.

Intravenous: 300 mg by infusion 6 hourly. Children 30–50 mg/kg/day in divided doses 6 hourly.

Chloramphenicol

Very effective broad-spectrum antibiotic but use is restricted because of bone marrow suppression, which occurs as a rare complication of treatment. Chloramphenicol is indicated in life-threatening infections for which other agents are unsuitable because of bacterial resistance or patient allergy. The drug is particularly useful in *H. influenzae* meningitis and typhoid fever. Chloramphenicol is contraindicated in neonates because of cardiovascular collapse (Chapter 3).

Dose

Intravenous: 1 g 6 hourly in adults. Children require 50–100 mg/kg daily divided in 6-hourly doses.

Fusidic acid

Narrow spectrum and indicated only in penicillin-resistant staphylococcal infections of bone.

Dose

500 mg 8 hourly by intravenous infusion or orally.

Clindamycin

Effective against penicillin-resistant staphylococci and many anaerobic organisms. However, a major adverse effect is pseudomembranous colitis caused by a toxin produced by *Clostridium difficile*, and clindamycin is indicated only in life-threatening infections where other agents are contraindicated.

Dose

0.6–2.7 g daily in divided doses by slow intravenous infusion. Children 15–40 mg/kg daily in divided doses.

Nitrofurantoin is effective against many organisms infecting the urinary tract, but it is a second-line drug for this indication because of frequent adverse effects including gastrointestinal symptoms and rashes. It precipitates haemolytic anaemia in glucose-6-phosphate deficiency and can cause peripheral neuropathy and pulmonary fibrosis.

Nalidixic acid is another urinary antimicrobial whose use is restricted by frequent adverse reactions.

Polymyxins are effective against *Pseudomonas* but frequent nephrotoxicity and the availability of safer, more effective drugs greatly limits use.

Vancomycin is effective against *Cl. difficile* when given orally and and is also used in prophylaxis of endocarditis caused by Gram-positive cocci.

9.3 ANTITUBERCULOUS DRUGS

Antituberculous drugs may be subdivided into three groups:
  (1) First line: isoniazid, rifampicin.
  (2) Second line: ethambutol, pyrazinamide, streptomycin.
  (3) Third line: capreomycin, cycloserine, ethionamide.

Isoniazid

Mechanism

The precise mechanism is unknown, but it is bactericidal.

Pharmacokinetics

Isoniazid is well absorbed following oral administration and is widely distributed including to the CSF where concentrations equal those in blood.

Isoniazid is inactivated in the liver by pathways including genetically-dependent acetylation. The same metabolic pathway is involved in the acetylation of hydralazine, procainamide and dapsone (Chapter 1.4). About 50% of the European and USA populations are slow acetylators but the proportion varies widely in other populations, and slow acetylation is very common in orientals.

Adverse effects

Peripheral neuropathy occurs mainly in slow acetylators and can be prevented by co-administration of pyridoxine (20 mg/day). Hepatotoxicity occasionally occurs and is more frequent in the elderly and those with a large alcohol intake. Very high doses of isoniazid can lead to psychosis, convulsions or coma.

Drug interactions

Inhibits enzymes which metabolise phenytoin and warfarin so phenytoin concentrations and anticoagulation level should be carefully monitored.

Dose

Oral: 3 mg/kg adults or 6 mg/kg daily in children, i.e. children require more on a weight basis. For tuberculous meningitis 10 mg/kg daily. Also available for parenteral use.

Rifampicin

Mechanism

It is bactericidal, and inhibits the DNA-dependent RNA polymerase of mycobacteria.

Pharmacokinetics

It is well absorbed following oral administration and widely distributed including to the CSF. Rifampicin is deacetylated in the liver and eliminated by biliary excretion.

Adverse effects

There is often a transient elevation of liver enzymes but serious hepatotoxicity is uncommon. The risk of liver damage is increased by alcoholism and pre-existing liver disease. Intermittent treatment is associated with more frequent and serious adverse effects including renal failure and thrombocytopaenia.

Drug interactions

Rifampicin induces hepatic enzymes and, because of increased clearance, can cause treatment failure with: oral contraceptives, sulphonylureas, warfarin, steroids and barbiturates.

Dose

10 mg/kg daily before breakfast.

Ethambutol

Mechanism

The mechanism is uncertain but bacteriostatic.

Pharmacokinetics

It is well absorbed following oral administration. It has poor penetration to CSF but otherwise is adequately distributed. Excretion of unchanged drug, is mainly renal.

Adverse effects

Most important reaction is retrobulbar neuritis with loss of visual acuity and colour vision. This is largely preventable by using doses below 25 mg/kg/day. The visual defect usually reverses over several months after stopping the drug.

Drug interactions

Aluminium hydroxide can decrease absorption.

Dose

15–25 mg/kg/day.

Pyrazinamide is bactericidal, penetrates the CSF very effectively and would be indicated in tuberculous meningitis. It is used in combination with rifampicin and isoniazid and is possibly more effective (and certainly cheaper) than ethambutol.

Streptomycin is now infrequently used. It is an aminoglycoside which is eliminated by the kidneys. Ototoxicity is the main adverse reaction. Streptomycin could particularly be considered for use in patients with liver disease.

Other antituberculous drugs. Several other agents are available for use in situations of bacterial resistance or adverse reactions to first or second-line drugs, e.g. capreomycin, cycloserine and ethionamide.

Comment

Tuberculous organisms multiply slowly and the long periods of treatment which are required encourage the emergence of resistant strains. Combination chemotherapy is thus the basis of treatment. Initially isoniazid, rifampicin and either ethambutol or pyrazinamide are administered for 8 weeks. Subsequently, isoniazid and rifampicin are given. Nine months treatment is adequate for pulmonary TB and 12 months for infection elsewhere.

9.4   ANTIFUNGAL DRUGS

Amphotericin B

Mechanism

It combines with sterols in plasma membrane with resulting increase in permeability and cell death.

Pharmacokinetics

Absorption is negligible following oral administration. In practice it is usually given intravenously. It is highly protein bound with apparently poor penetration to tissues and body fluids. It is not removed by haemodialysis. Mode of elimination is unknown but not influenced by renal function.

Adverse effects

These are very common. Most patients develop fever, chills and nausea. Nephrotoxicity (distal tubular destruction and calcification) usually occurs during prolonged treatment at or above 1 mg/kg day and manifests as hypokalaemia, loss of concentrating ability and renal tubular acidosis. Reverses if detected early.

Drug interaction

Additive with other nephrotoxic drugs. Concurrent digoxin therapy can become toxic if hypokalaemia develops.

Antifungal spectrum

Currently drug of choice for most systemic mycoses: active against *Cryptococcus*, *Candida* and other yeasts, *Aspergillus*, *Coccidioides* and other fungi. Resistance has not been reported.

Dose

1 mg test dose. Then 250 μg/kg daily increasing to 1–1.5 mg daily depending on disease severity and appearance of nephrotoxicity.

Hydrocortisone can reduce febrile reactions and chlorpromazine can reduce nausea.

Comment

Amphotericin B is an example of risks and benefits of treatment having to be carefully weighed. It is highly toxic but systemic mycoses are frequently fatal.

Flucytosine

Mechanism

It is deaminated inside fungal cell to 5-fluorouracil which inhibits nucleic acid synthesis with cell death.

Pharmacokinetics

It is well absorbed following oral administration and is widely distributed including the CSF. Elimination is mainly renal. Clearance is decreased in patients with renal impairment.

Adverse effects

Concentration related bone marrow suppression is the only major problem. This can usually be avoided by drug level monitoring.

Antifungal spectrum

Only active against yeasts, but efficacy limited by resistance.

Dose

150–200 mg daily in divided doses.

Comment

Although much less toxic than amphotericin, flucytosine is of limited value because of its narrow spectrum and the existence of resistant organisms.

Miconazole, clotrimazole, econazole, ketoconazole

Mechanism

Increase permeability by preventing ergosterol formation in cell membrane. Also produce cell necrosis by inhibiting peroxidative enzymes.

Pharmacokinetics

Poorly absorbed following oral administration except ketoconazole. These drugs are widely distributed except to CSF. Eliminated by hepatic metabolism.

Adverse effects

Relatively mild: deranged liver function tests, nausea and occasionally confusion; all reversible.

Antifungal spectrum

Wide range of yeasts and fungi. Main use at present is topical, e.g. athlete's foot or vaginal candidiasis. However, intravenous miconazole is indicated in patients who cannot tolerate amphotericin and ketoconazole is effective in chronic mucocutaneous candidosis and possibly in other fungal infections.

Dose

Miconazole: 600 mg 8 hourly intravenously.
Ketoconazole: 200–400 mg orally as single daily dose.

Nystatin is used topically in the treatment of yeast infections of the skin and mucous membranes. It is not used parenterally because of high toxicity.

Griseofulvin is active only against dermatophytes and is given orally in the treatment of skin or nail infections. It is fungistatic so must be given for weeks or months. It diminishes anticoagulant effect by enzyme induction. Barbiturates lead to griseofulvin treatment failure by enzyme induction. Griseofulvin can precipitate porphyria.

9.5   ANTIVIRAL DRUGS

These are the least developed group of antimicrobial agents: viruses utilise the biochemical systems of their host cell, and it is therefore very difficult to prevent viral multiplication without seriously damaging the patient.

Idoxuridine

Idoxuridine is a thymidine analogue which inhibits DNA synthesis. It is highly toxic when given systemically and is only used topically in the treatment of herpes simplex infections of the eye, skin and genitalia.

Vidarabine

Vidarabine also inhibits DNA synthesis. It is used systemically in the treatment of chicken pox or herpes zoster infections in immunocompromised hosts. In addition, it decreases the early mortality in herpes simplex encephalitis. The major adverse reactions are suppression of bone marrow and a wide range of neurological signs.

Amantadine

Amantadine prevents entry of influenza A to host cells and can be prophylactic against infections caused by this virus. It can produce neurological effects but these are usually seen only if high concentrations are achieved, e.g. in renal failure.

Acyclovir

Acyclovir is preferentially absorbed by herpes infected cells and then phosphorylated by a herpes specified enzyme to a compound which has considerably greater activity against viral compared to human DNA. Effective topically against herpetic ulcers. When given intravenously it is effective prophylaxis against herpes infections in immunocompromised hosts. Appears to be less toxic than earlier antiviral drugs.

CHAPTER 10

Drugs and respiratory disease

10.1   Drugs and airflow obstruction

10.2   Oxygen

10.3   Respiratory stimulants

10.4   Expectorants and cough suppressants

10.1   DRUGS AND AIRFLOW OBSTRUCTION

Aims

The aim of treatment in airflow obstruction is to increase ventilation by reducing bronchial smooth muscle tone with specific agonist and antagonist drugs and by blocking the mechanisms of the allergic response.

Relevant pathophysiology

The efficiency of carbon dioxide and oxygen exchange in the alveoli of the lungs depends on many factors including:
  (1) Alveolar ventilation,
  (2) Pulmonary blood flow,
  (3) The matching of ventilation and perfusion,
  (4) The quantity of haemoglobin in the blood and its affinity for oxygen.
  Alveolar   ventilation   is   controlled   by   chemoreceptor, mechanoreceptor   and   other   reflex   mechanisms.   The   autonomic

139

nervous system is an important regulator of smooth muscle tone in the small airways which is the main factor determining airflow resistance. Bronchial smooth muscle tone is regulated by:

(1) Parasympathetic constrictor effects mediated by vagal muscarinic cholinergic receptors.

(2) Adrenergic bronchodilator effects mediated by adrenoceptors of the $beta_2$-type innervated by sympathetic nerves or responding to circulating catecholamines. $Beta_2$-receptor stimulation activates adenyl cyclase and increases intracellular cyclic AMP.

(3) Other humoral agents which increase bronchomotor tone include histamine, serotonin, bradykinin, slow-reacting substance of anaphylaxis and eosinophil chemotactic factor. These agents may reach the lungs as circulating humoral factors or be released from sensitised mast cells in the lung itself when mast cells, with IgE antibody bound to the surface, are exposed to a specific antigen (Type I hypersensitivity, Chapter 12.2) as occurs in allergic or extrinsic asthma. Mast cells are stabilised by $beta_2$-receptor stimulants and other agents.

There are two common conditions when bronchomotor tone is pathologically disturbed: (1) asthma, and (2) chronic obstructive airways disease (or chronic bronchitis and emphysema).

Asthma is a reversible increase in airways resistance or bronchial tone. It may be exercise induced or related to specific extrinsic allergens. *Extrinsic asthma*, which characteristically begins in childhood, is associated with eczema or hay fever. Hypersensitivity to specific allergens by inhalation or skin testing can be demonstrated. Increased levels of allergen specific IgE antibody are found in plasma and bronchial constriction results from a Type I hypersensitivity reaction. *Intrinsic asthma*, which also shows a reversible component, usually develops later in life and has no readily identifiable precipitating factors or allergens.

Chronic obstructive airways disease is usually associated with cigarette smoking and is characterised by increased sputum production and cough for many years. Airways obstruction is often only partly reversible and in many cases irreversible obstruction with lung destruction caused by emphysema is found.

This classification is not exclusive and many patients do not readily fit into a single category. Of more importance is the functional assessment of response to bronchodilator drugs using test doses and measurement of the improvement in expiratory gas flow.

Drugs used in the treatment of airways obstruction

The main groups of drugs used in airflow obstruction are:

(1) Beta$_2$-adrenoceptor agonists or stimulants, which increase cyclic AMP in bronchial muscle cells and mast cells.

(2) Theophylline and other xanthine derivatives, which block phosphodiesterase and thereby also increase intracellular cyclic AMP.

(3) Mast cell membrane stabilisers like sodium cromoglycate, which prevent release of bronchoconstrictor mediators.

(4) Corticosteroids, which may stabilise mast cells and improve pulmonary function in extrinsic and intrinsic asthma by other unidentified mechanisms.

(5) Anticholinergic (muscarinic) drugs, which reduce cholinergic bronchoconstriction.

Beta$_2$-adrenoceptor agonists

Salbutamol

Mechanism

Agents such as salbutamol, terbutaline and fenoterol are selective stimulants of beta$_2$-adrenoceptors. They act on beta$_2$-receptors in the bronchi and small airways and on mast cells. They cause fewer cardiac beta$_1$ effects than adrenaline or isoprenaline, which are non-selective and can be regarded as obsolete.

The main actions of beta$_2$-agonists are:

(1) Relaxation of bronchial smooth muscle,

(2) Stabilising mast cells.

Both actions are mediated by increased intracellular cyclic AMP. Salbutamol like other beta$_2$-stimulants is best given by inhalation as this permits delivery of the drug directly to the site of action and reduces the possibility of generalised systemic effects. The total dose administered by aerosol is very much lower than by mouth, further limiting dose-related adverse effects. Salbutamol has a relatively long duration of action of 4 h or longer.

Adverse effects

Salbutamol may cause tremor by stimulation of $beta_2$-receptors. Other dose dependent adverse effects which result from weak $beta_1$-activity include tachycardia and hypokalaemia. These are rare, however, with the higher degree of selectivity afforded by the aerosol route of administration.

Clinical use and dose

Used in asthma and chronic obstructive airways disease in long-term prophylactic or maintenance therapy (aerosol or oral tablets) or in acute attacks by nebuliser.

By aerosol inhalation: 0.1–0.2 mg four to six times daily.

By nebuliser: 2 ml of a 0.5% solution four times daily or 1–2 mg/h.

By mouth: 2–4 mg three or four times daily.

Salbutamol may also be given by intravenous injection.

Terbutaline and Fenoterol

These are other selective $beta_2$-stimulants with actions very similar to salbutamol. They are available as oral, parenteral and inhalational preparations and their adverse effects and indications are also similar to those for salbutamol.

Other selective beta$_2$-stimulants

A number of alternative $beta_2$-agonists are available including isoetharine, rimiterol and reproterol. These agents are either less selective or shorter acting and have no clear advantages over salbutamol or terbutaline. Their indications and adverse effects are described above.

Comment

Beta$_2$-adrenoceptor agonists given by aerosol inhalation result in symptomatic relief with minimal cardiac adverse effects in many patients with reversible airways obstruction. Response depends on the patient using the aerosol correctly. Even with optimal use, only about 10% of the drug is inhaled. The rest is swallowed.

Theophylline

Mechanism

Theophylline and other xanthine derivatives are phosphodiesterase inhibitors. They increase cyclic AMP concentrations by blocking the enzyme phosphodiesterase, which usually breaks down the nucleotide. Increased cyclic AMP reduces tone in bronchial smooth muscle and stabilises mast cell membranes. Xanthines may have widespread effects on smooth muscle not only in the bronchi but also in the cardiovascular system.

Pharmacokinetics

Theophylline is well absorbed from the gut. It is extensively metabolised by the liver and differences in hepatic metabolism are the principal reason for the wide variation in kinetics, both between individuals and within the same individual during the course of an illness (Chapter 5.2). There is a well-defined relationship between concentration and effect. The degree of bronchodilatation increases linearly with the plasma concentration. However, the response varies from individual to individual. The maximum response may be limited by structural damage to the airways in chronic bronchitis and emphysema or by adverse effects at plasma concentrations above 25 µg/ml. The average elimination half-life in adults is about 8–12 h. Theophylline is therefore given orally two or three times daily. The dosage schedules depend on the assessment of clearance in individual patients. In children and young adults theophylline clearance is considerably increased requiring a higher daily dose. In the elderly, particularly those with congestive cardiac failure or respiratory failure, theophylline clearance may be correspondingly reduced with lower dose requirements (Chapter 3.4 and Chapter 5).

Adverse effects

Tachycardia, palpitation, nausea, vomiting and convulsions are associated with plasma levels above 25–30 µg/ml. Nausea may occur at therapeutic plasma levels.

Clinical use and dose

Theophylline is used orally in the long-term treatment of asthma and chronic obstructive airways disease in those patients who show a response to it. Several tablet formulations are available. The dose should be adjusted using therapeutic response, adverse effects and, if available, plasma level measurements. The dose ranges from 200–600 mg two or three times daily. Theophylline is equally effective as a suppository.

Aminophylline contains theophylline and ethylenediamine (2 : 1). It can be given orally (450–1250 mg/day in divided doses) or by suppository. Aminophylline is also used intravenously in the treatment of:

(1) Severe acute attacks of asthma (status asthmaticus),

(2) Exacerbations of chronic obstructive airways disease,

(3) Acute left ventricular failure with pulmonary oedema.

A loading dose of 6 mg/kg (250–500 mg) is given over 10–20 min intravenously. Intravenous infusion (0.5–0.9 mg/kg/h) may be continued, but it is advisable to obtain plasma level measurements if the infusion is maintained for more than 4–6 h.

Comment

Oral theophylline preparations are useful in the long-term treatment of asthma and the reversible component of chronic obstructive airways disease. A useful bronchodilator response can often be achieved within the therapeutic range and adverse effects can be minimised with the aid of plasma level measurements.

Beta$_2$-adrenoceptor agonists and theophylline preparations reduce bronchial tone and stabilise mast cells by increasing intracellular cyclic AMP by different mechanisms. Oral theophylline and beta$_2$-agonists are widely used together. However, the optimum combination dose has not yet been established.

Mast cell stabilisers

Sodium cromoglycate and ketotifen

Mechanism

These drugs are *not* bronchodilators but prevent bronchoconstriction in patients with extrinsic or allergic asthma.

They stabilise sensitised mast cells and inhibit the release of bronchoconstrictor agents including histamine, serotonin and slow-reacting substance (Chapter 12.2).

Mast cell stabilisers are useful in extrinsic (allergic) asthma, particularly in children and young adults and can prevent exercise-induced asthma. Response in intrinsic asthma is usually disappointing and these agents have nothing to offer patients with chronic obstructive airways disease.

Clinical use and dose

Sodium cromoglycate is administered locally to the lungs by inhalation as a powder (20 mg two to eight times daily) or from a pressurised aerosol or nebuliser (10 mg up to six times daily).

Ketotifen has not been evaluated so extensively as sodium cromoglycate. It is given orally as tablets or capsules 1–2 mg daily. Sedation and dry mouth may result from additional antihistamine effects of this drug.

Corticosteroids

The actions of corticosteroids on the bronchi are not fully understood. They have many actions which may contribute:
(1) Anti-inflammatory activity,
(2) Reduction of mucosal oedema,
(3) Modification of immune responses and mast cell stabilisation,
(4) Increased beta-adrenoceptor responsiveness to agonists.

The actions of corticosteroids and their adverse effects are discussed in Chapter 13.1.

In the management of airways obstruction, corticosteroids can be given by three routes:
(1) Inhalation,
(2) Orally,
(3) Intravenously.

Inhalation

Steroid aerosols represent a significant advance in the management of bronchospasm because adverse effects associated with systemic steroids are minimised. Beclomethasone and betamethasone are administered by aerosol inhalation, (100 μg, three or four times daily).

Adverse effects of inhaled steroids are usually very much less than those of systemic agents but infection of the pharynx and larynx with candidiasis may occur.

Comment

Aerosol inhalation of corticosteroids should replace long-term oral corticosteroid therapy wherever possible as the benefits can be obtained without the adverse consequences of long-term systemic steroid treatment.

Intravenous corticosteroids

In severe unresponsive asthma with respiratory failure hydrocortisone is given intravenously (100–200 mg or more). The dose can be repeated 4 hourly, but it is important to note that there is a delay in the onset of any steroid-induced bronchodilator effect and other measures should be pursued aggressively at the same time.

Oral corticosteroids

Patients with severe exacerbations of asthma require high doses of prednisolone by mouth after intravenous hydrocortisone. Steroids are started at 80 mg/day of prednisolone for 1–2 days and reduced over the next 4–6 days to 10–15 mg/day after which inhaled steroids may be substituted.

Anticholinergic drugs

Mechanism

The parasympathetic cholinergic bronchoconstrictor effect can be blocked by atropine-like drugs. Usually this effect of anticholinergics on airway resistance is less than that of the sympathetic agents. The anticholinergic adverse effects (Chapter 19.2) of the synthetic derivative, ipratropium bromide, are much less than those of atropine itself. It is given as 18–36 μg three or four times daily by pressurised aerosol or from a nebuliser.

The management of airways obstruction

Asthma

Patients with allergic extrinsic asthma should avoid known allergens and may benefit from desensitisation. Sodium cromoglycate or ketotifen or topical steroid can be used prophylactically. If functional impairment persists a beta$_2$-receptor agonist by aerosol or theophylline or both may be required depending on the severity of symptoms. If in exacerbation of asthma symptoms are not improved within a few hours the condition is called status asthmaticus and requires emergency hospital admission for intensive treatment.

Status asthmaticus

(1) Clinical assessment may be misleading. Repeated blood gas measurements and simple pulmonary function tests should be used to assess the severity of the attack and the response to treatment.

(2) High concentration oxygen therapy is indicated since hypoxia is acute.

(3) Aerosol beta$_2$-agonist can be conveniently added from a nebuliser in the oxygen flow. This route is probably preferable to the intravenous one.

(4) Intravenous aminophylline as a loading dose, followed by an intravenous infusion, may be used.

(5) Intravenous hydrocortisone followed by a course of high dose oral steroids may be required.

(6) If the exacerbation was preceded by an upper respiratory tract infection then appropriate antibiotics should be given after sputum has been collected for culture.

(7) Intravenous fluids should be given as dehydration contributes to the clinical features of status asthmaticus.

(8) Sedatives, anxiolytics, opiate analgesics and hypnotics should *not* be used as central depression of ventilation may worsen respiratory failure.

(9) Artificial ventilation may be required if respiratory failure, exhaustion of the respiratory muscles or circulatory collapse occur.

Comment

Asthma is a serious condition whose severity is difficult to assess clinically and may be life threatening. Failure to respond to the patient's usual treatment is an indication for aggressive intervention with careful monitoring of ventilatory function.

Chronic obstructive airways disease

(1) Patients should stop smoking.

(2) If pulmonary function tests indicate a reversible component to beta$_2$-agonist or anticholinergic drugs these should be given by aerosol.

(3) In patients who can be shown to respond to it, oral theophylline with therapeutic monitoring of plasma levels should be used alone or together with the agents above.

(4) Intercurrent chest infections are associated with acute exacerbations and should be treated with antibiotics guided by sputum culture and with physiotherapy.

(5) If heart failure (cor pulmonale) develops diuretic therapy is indicated. Venesection may be indicated for the secondary polycythaemia which is often associated.

(6) Patients with severe chronic obstructive airways disease who develop respiratory failure should have oxygen therapy at low ·concentration, physiotherapy to assist expectoration and ventilation.

10.2   OXYGEN

When oxygen is given to supplement the amount normally present in inspired air it should be regarded as a drug. Oxygen is given either:

(1) In as high a concentration as possible, or

(2) In low (24–28%) controlled concentrations.

High oxygen concentrations

High oxygen concentrations should be given to all hypoxic patients except those with established or potential CO_2 narcosis. Any apparatus which provides an oxygen flow to the oronasal area at a rate of 5 l/min or more is effective in supplying a high concentration of oxygen in the inspired gas. Masks with a dead-space volume under 100 ml do not cause carbon dioxide rebreathing; nasal cannulae cause none at all.

Indications for high oxygen concentrations include:
 (1) Pneumonia,
 (2) Acute pulmonary oedema,
 (3) Pulmonary thromboembolism,
 (4) Fibrosing alveolitis,
 (5) Status asthmaticus,
 (6) Acute respiratory failure or arrest (e.g. due to drug overdose),
 (7) Acute circulatory failure,
 (8) Severe anaemia,
 (9) Cyanide and carbon monoxide poisoning.

Low (controlled) oxygen concentrations

Low concentration oxygen therapy is reserved for patients with exacerbations of chronic obstructive airways disease with respiratory failure. Ventilation is then so ineffective that carbon dioxide excretion is not maintained in spite of a raised arterial P_{CO_2}. The increased P_{CO_2} leads to loss of sensitivity of the respiratory centre to CO_2 and a dependence on low arterial P_{O_2} to drive ventilation. High concentration oxygen administration leads to further suppression of ventilation by removal of the hypoxic drive. Further carbon dioxide accumulation then rapidly produces narcosis and death.

Low concentrations may be administered by masks using the venturi principle to supply a calibrated inspired O_2 concentration of 24 or 28%.

10.3   RESPIRATORY STIMULANTS

Some patients with respiratory failure require intubation and artificial ventilation. The place of respiratory stimulants is controversial. They may occasionally lead to an improvement in ventilation and obviate the need for assisted respiration.

Nikethamide

Nikethamide is a convulsant or analeptic used in subconvulsant doses. Its central activating effect is not selective for the respiratory centre. Its effects are transient, lasting about 5 min. Adverse effects include vomiting, restlessness and convulsions. This drug may be used in respiratory depression following inappropriate oxygen therapy in doses of 0.5–2 g intravenously repeated after 10–20 min.

Doxapram

Doxapram is also an analeptic but is given by continuous intravenous infusion. It is used in doses of 1–4 mg/min to stimulate respiration in patients who fail to ventilate spontaneously after general anaesthesia and in chronic respiratory failure with carbon dioxide retention.

10.4 EXPECTORANTS AND COUGH SUPPRESSANTS

Two other classes of drugs, expectorants and cough suppressants, are commonly used in respiratory disease but their therapeutic value is doubtful.

Expectorants

Difficulty in bringing up sputum is a common complaint, but there is no evidence that any agent given by any route specifically promoted expectoration of bronchial secretions. Nevertheless, agents with 'expectorant' properties, ammonium chloride and guaiphenesin, are often included in proprietary cough mixtures. Agents claimed to possess mucolytic properties such as acetyl cysteine have not been conclusively shown to have an important role in the management of airways obstruction. Their beneficial effect may be attributed to the inhalation of steam or water by aerosol rather than the pharmacological properties of the drugs concerned.

Cough suppressants

Cough is a frequent complaint often secondary to an upper respiratory tract infection. Chronic persistent cough is often caused by cigarette smoking. In acute respiratory infections cough is a useful protective mechanism enabling the clearing of secretion from the trachea and bronchi. Cough usually improves spontaneously with treatment of any underlying bacterial infection. Patients with terminal lung cancer with bronchial obstruction or tumour involvement of afferent sensory nerves from the lung and chest wall may develop a persistent distressing cough. This is one of the few conditions in which symptomatic treatment of cough can be completely justified.

Cough suppressants are opiate agonists and the suppression of cough reflexes is only part of the narcotic induced depression of the central nervous system (Chapter 17).

The following drugs are used for cough suppression usually in the form of a sweet syrup or linctus (although oral or parenteral opiate will block cough reflexes just as effectively).

Diamorphine (linctus, 3 mg/5 ml)
Methadone (linctus, 2 mg/5 ml)
Codeine (linctus, 15 mg/5 ml).

CHAPTER 11

Drugs and rheumatic disease

11.1 Principles of drug treatment

11.2 Simple analgesics and non-steroidal anti-inflammatory drugs

11.3 Second- and third-line drugs in arthritis

11.4 Drugs used in gout

Aims

In inflammatory joint disease, the aims are:
(1) To reduce pain,
(2) To reduce stiffness and improve mobility,
(3) To prevent chronic deformity by minimising the inflammation which results in synovial membrane proliferation and bone erosions.

Relevant pathophysiology

Anti-inflammatory analgesic drugs are used to relieve the painful symptoms of joint diseases, including:
Rheumatoid arthritis,
Osteoarthritis,
Ankylosing spondylitis,
Gout,
Arthritis associated with Reiter's Syndrome,
Arthritis associated with systemic lupus erythematosis.
The aetiology of these diseases is varied and in most cases not entirely clear, but with the exception of gout and possibly

osteoarthritis there seems to be a disturbance in immune responses. In rheumatoid arthritis, for example, immune complexes composed of immunoglobulins of the IgM type activate complement and release factors which are chemotactic for neutrophil polymorphs. Released lysosomal enzymes damage cartilage while prostaglandins promote synovial vasodilatation and exacerbate pain. Thus there are a number of areas where an anti-inflammatory drug might be effective:

(1) Immunosuppression,
(2) Inhibition of cell migration,
(3) Inhibition of enzyme release,
(4) Inhibition of prostaglandin synthesis.

The most potent agents used in rheumatoid arthritis are gold, d-penicillamine and corticosteroids, but they have major problems associated with their long-term use and are therefore reserved for second- or third-line treatment. Initially, symptoms are treated with non-steroidal anti-inflammatory drugs. Aspirin, first commercially prepared by Felix Hofmann in 1893, is still widely used and the standard by which newer agents are judged.

11.1 PRINCIPLES OF DRUG TREATMENT

While drugs are an important part of the treatment of patients with inflammatory joint disease such as rheumatoid arthritis, other aspects demand careful consideration. These include rest, exercise and psychological management.

Rest

Rheumatoid arthritis is typically a disease of exacerbation and remission. During an acute attack it may be necessary to recommend bed rest, with local support and splinting of the affected joints.

Exercise

After an acute attack, carefully graded exercises are required to ensure an early return to normal activities. Either excessive rest or excessive exercise can be harmful.

Psychological management

The patient should be sympathetically introduced to the view that the disease has no ultimate cure. Acute onset and early remission are favourable signs, while an insidious onset, gradual deterioration with no remission over a year herald an unfavourable prognosis.

Various physical aids are available to make domestic life easier for the more severely affected patient. Some forms of physical therapy such as wax baths and hydrotherapy may be helpful.

11.2 SIMPLE ANALGESICS AND NON-STEROIDAL ANTI-INFLAMMATORY DRUGS

Simple analgesics

Simple analgesics such as paracetamol may be used to supplement other therapy, but they are relatively ineffective when used singly in rheumatoid arthritis. They do nothing to retard the progress of the disease and cannot provide adequate pain relief. They may be adequate in the management of some patients with osteoarthritis.

Non-steroidal anti-inflammatory drugs (NSAIDs)

The mechanism of action of NSAIDs is unknown. Many effects have been found *in vitro*, but their correlation with clinical efficacy is poor. All are inhibitors of prostaglandin synthesis, either cyclooxygenase or lipooxygenase inhibitors. Lysosome-stabilising effects and inhibition of cellular migration have also been demonstrated but, again, the clinical significance of this observation is unclear.

Aspirin and related compounds

Aspirin is the longest established anti-inflammatory drug. Its efficacy was emphasised in a study of 300 patients with rheumatoid arthritis in which 20% were chair or bed bound at the start of the study. About a year later only 15% were confined to chair or bed and 60% were living independently. Treatment consisted exclusively of rest, splinting, physiotherapy and aspirin. Set against the natural history of rheumatoid arthritis these are impressive figures. In addition, aspirin is relatively cheap. Tablets of 300 mg even in enteric-coated form may cost only one-tenth of the newer propionic acid derivatives.

Pharmacokinetics

The pharmacokinetics of aspirin are complex and when used in relatively high dose for long periods of time plasma levels should be monitored. Aspirin is readily absorbed from the gastrointestinal tract and is given orally. Elimination varies from individual to individual. Clearance is dose dependent like that of phenytoin reflecting zero-order elimination (Chapter 5.2).

Adverse effects

Gastrointestinal effects. Nausea and vomiting follow high doses of aspirin. Dyspepsia, gastric irritation and occult or frank blood loss are common adverse effects particularly when aspirin is associated with alcohol ingestion. Blood loss results from superficial gastric erosions or peptic ulceration. Inhibition of prostaglandin synthesis is probably responsible for some prostaglandins increase gastric mucosal blood flow and have other protective effects. Gastrointestinal blood loss occurs even with parenteral aspirin or preparations by suppository. However, fewer erosions and ulcers are found with these and more recent enteric-coated formulations. Newer NSAIDs have been claimed to cause less gastric irritation. These comparisons have not usually been made with enteric-coated aspirin. At present there appears to be a dose-dependent relationship between anti-inflammatory analgesic effect, prostaglandin synthetase inhibition and the frequency of gastric irritation. Less active analgesics cause less gastric irritation.

Prolonged bleeding time may result from inhibition of thromboxane synthesis and impaired platelet aggregation (Chapter 16.5) or reduced hepatic clotting factor synthesis.

Bronchospasm, urticaria or hay fever rarely may occur in sensitive individuals and appear to result from release of immune mediators secondary to prostaglandin synthesis inhibition.

Tinnitus, dizziness and deafness are dose and plasma level related adverse effects. Vomiting and tachypnoea may also occur.

In *overdose* confusion, convulsions and hyperpyrexia are seen. Forced diuresis may speed elimination of aspirin in cases of poisoning (Chapter 21.2).

Dose

Aspirin tablets, 300–900 mg 4–6 hourly. In rheumatoid arthritis, up to 4.2 g/day may be required in divided doses.

Phenylbutazone

Phenylbutazone is a potent anti-inflammatory agent. Its use is now limited to acute gout and ankylosing spondylitis.

Pharmacokinetics

Phenylbutazone is an acidic drug that is rapidly absorbed from the gastrointestinal tract. It is extensively bound to plasma proteins and is metabolised in the liver. One of its metabolites, oxyphenbutazone, also has anti-inflammatory activity.

Adverse effects

Phenylbutazone shares with aspirin a high incidence of gastric intolerance. It also has sodium-retaining properties and may precipitate cardiac failure in elderly subjects. Phenylbutazone may cause a drug-induced hepatitis. Blood dyscrasias present the most serious life-threatening adverse effect. Agranulocytosis, seen early in the course of treatment of younger subjects, is often reversed on stopping the drug, but aplastic anaemia, developing after months or years in older subjects is frequently fatal. The incidence of aplastic anaemia is low but such a potentially fatal complication of treatment for a disease that is generally non-fatal is unacceptable. There is no justification now for the long-term use of phenylbutazone although it may be used in short-term treatment particularly in gouty arthritis where an additional benefit is derived from its uricosuric effect.

Drug interactions

Phenylbutazone, which is extensively protein bound and metabolised by the liver, has a high potential for interaction with drugs which share these properties. Phenylbutazone and the oral anticoagulant warfarin interact and the overall effect is to enhance anticoagulant activity, giving rise to a haemorrhagic diathesis (Chapter 16.5). Phenylbutazone in the short term displaces warfarin from binding sites and in the longer term inhibits hepatic metabolism of warfarin (Chapter 1.4).

Indomethacin and related drugs

Indomethacin has been widely used in inflammatory joint disease for years. It is given by mouth and by suppository. Gastric adverse effects are a predictable problem, but headache, mental confusion and dizziness may also present problems. Salt and water retention with oedema may aggravate cardiac failure or hypertension and reduce the efficacy of antihypertensive drugs. Rectal administration may be associated with pruritis, discomfort and bleeding.

Dose

Orally, 25–50 mg, 2–3 times daily
Rectally by suppository, 100 mg at night; this may be repeated in the morning.
   Sulindac is similar to indomethacin. It is a pro-drug which is inactive in the stomach and may show reduced gastric intolerance. It is converted to its active form by hydrolysis after absorption.

Propionic acid derivatives

A large number of agents from this group of drugs has been marketed recently. They are well absorbed orally, and have fewer gastric adverse effects than plain aspirin. This has led some rheumatologists to favour them as first-line therapy. This group consists of the following drugs:
   Ibuprofen,
   Fenoprofen,
   Ketoprofen,
   Naproxen,

Flurbiprofen,
Fenbufen,
Benoxaprofen.

Fenbufen is also a pro-drug with no direct anti-inflammatory activity in the stomach.

Benoxaprofen has lipooxygenase-inhibiting activity, but inhibits cellular migration in animal models. It has a long half-life and is given once a day.

None of these propionic acid derivatives has been shown to interact significantly with oral anticoagulants, and if a patient must also receive warfarin, this group of drugs is preferable.

Phenylacetic acid derivatives

Diclofenac and fenclofenac are very similar to the propionic acid derivatives.

Fenclofenac has a high incidence of drug rash which appears early in the course of treatment and disappears rapidly when the drug is stopped. It may reduce ESR and rheumatoid factor titre.

Diclofenac is less liable to produce a rash.

Fenamates

The long established mefenamic acid and flufenamic acid are effective in inflammatory joint disease, but they share the problems of salicylates to which they are chemically related. Thus, they share the gastric adverse effects of other anti-inflammatory drugs but, in addition, they cause diarrhoea, a dose-related phenomenon, the basis of which is not clear.

Piroxicam

This is a new anti-inflammatory agent, chemically unrelated to other drugs. It does, however, share their propensity to cause gastrointestinal adverse effects, and potentiates the effect of oral anticoagulants. It is also contraindicated in asthmatic patients who cannot tolerate aspirin.

Comment

This group of drugs forms the first line and mainstay of treatment of inflammatory arthritis. There is now a bewildering array of strongly promoted agents. Despite this, no one drug has been shown to be clearly superior to the remainder in terms of symptomatic relief, disease suppression or toxic effects. It is advisable to become familiar with a few drugs and restrict use to these. Unfortunately, individual response to a particular drug is somewhat unpredictable and the choice of drug is inescapably empirical. A list of the principal NSAIDs and their doses is presented in Table 11.1.

TABLE 11.1 Examples of the principal groups of non-steroidal anti-inflammatory drugs.

Drug	Typical dosage schedule	
SALICYLATES		
Aspirin	900 mg	4–hourly*
Diflunisal	500 mg	12–hourly
Benorylate	4 g	12–hourly
PYRAZOLES		
Phenylbutazone	100 mg	8–hourly
Azapropazone	300 mg	6–hourly
INDOLES		
Indomethacin	50 mg	8–hourly
Sulindac	200 mg	12–hourly
FENAMATES		
Mefenamic acid	500 mg	8–hourly
Flufenamic acid	200 mg	8–hourly
PROPIONATES		
Ibuprofen	400 mg	8–hourly
Naproxen	250 mg	8–hourly
Ketoprofen	50 mg	6–hourly
PHENYLACETATES		
Diclofenac	50 mg	8–hourly
OTHER		
Piroxicam	20 mg	daily

* Adjust according to serum concentration.
These dose schedules are near the upper limit and therapy should be commenced with approximately half doses.

11.3 SECOND- AND THIRD-LINE DRUGS IN ARTHRITIS

These anti-rheumatic agents comprise a group of widely different chemical entities including gold, penicillamine, chloroquine and, more recently sulphasalazine, levamisole and dapsone. Corticosteroids and immunosuppressant cytotoxic drugs are used as third-line therapy.

Mechanisms of action of second-line drugs are not clear. There is a lag between starting therapy and observing an effect. It is usual to continue with conventional anti-inflammatory drugs. These drugs, unlike most NSAIDs, may influence the underlying disease process. Haemoglobin may rise, ESR and rheumatoid factor titre may fall in patients who respond.

Gold salts

These have been used for over 40 years in the management of rheumatoid arthritis. Gold salts reduce macrophage activity. One-third of patients derive considerable benefit, one-third have only a modest response, and one-third have adverse effects and require interruption of treatment.

Adverse effects

(1) Pruritic rashes are common and present in many forms including mouth ulcers. Rashes are not always dose related and may not limit further gold use.

(2) Proteinuria secondary to a membranous glomerulonephritis occurs in 10% of patients. It resolves on stopping gold treatment.

(3) Vasodilatation with orthostatic hypotension may acutely follow drug dosing.

(4) Neutropenia, thrombocytopenia and aplastic anaemia are rare nowadays as gold treatment is closely supervised with weekly haematological checks. If white cell count or platelet count begins to fall treatment is interrupted.

Clinical use and dose

Intramuscular injection of sodium aurothiomalate 1, 5 and 10 mg at weekly intervals and then 50 mg weekly for up to 3 months or until a response or toxic effects are observed. Dose frequency may be reduced to monthly and continued for years. Gold is indicated in rheumatoid arthritis and also in psoriatic arthropathy.

d-Penicillamine

First introduced as a copper chelating agent in Wilson's disease, d-penicillamine modifies formation of immunoglobulin. It has a similar action to gold salts but relapse may occur with continuing therapy.

Adverse effects

These are similar to those with gold. Cross toxicity with gold has been reported but is disputed. It is likely that both gold and penicillamine toxicity are associated with the same HLA tissue type (DW3).

(1) Skin rashes are common,

(2) Proteinuria as with gold,

(3) Marrow toxicity is similar to gold consisting of thrombocytopenia and neutropenia. As these changes develop gradually, routine weekly haematological monitoring is essential.

(4) Immunological effects. Up to 50% of patients develop positive anti-nuclear factor tests. Systemic lupus erythematosus or myasthenia gravis may be precipitated.

Clinical use and dose

Penicillamine 125–250 mg daily increasing after 4–6 weeks to 250–500 mg daily.

Useful in rheumatoid arthritis and scleroderma.

Chloroquine and hydroxychloroquine

In rheumatoid arthritis, the mechanisms of action of these preparations, originally developed as antimalarials, may be by reducing ' T helper' lymphocytes and lysosome stabilisation.

They are well absorbed orally, taken up by many tissues and then very slowly excreted in the urine. The most disturbing toxic effects are opthalmological. An early keratitis is reversible but gradual accumulation of the drug in the retina can lead to irreversible retinal damage with permanent blindness after 1 year. Rashes and marrow toxicity are rarely seen. Neuropathies and myopathies have been reported.

Clinical use

Chloroquine is often given in interrupted courses with drug free periods of 2–3 months each year. Combination with D-penicillamine has proved useful. Chloroquine may be used in systemic lupus erythematosus as well as rheumatoid arthritis.

Levamisole

This drug stimulates depressed T-lymphocyte function (Chapter 12.2). It may cause rashes, gastrointestinal upset and agranulocytosis. The role of levamisole in rheumatoid arthritis and other immunological diseases is still controversial. Levamisole is given once or twice weekly with weekly white cell counts.

Corticosteroids

Corticosteroids have potent immunosuppressant activity (Chapter 12.2) and a range of other effects (Chapter 13). They are the most powerful anti-inflammatory drugs available.

In rheumatoid arthritis there is little evidence that high doses are more effective than low doses. For chronic use not more than 7.5 mg prednisolone per day or the equivalent can be given without the development of the spectrum of adverse effects (Chapter 13.1). Steroids are particularly useful in systemic lupus erythematosus and polymyalgia rheumatica.

Where one or two joints are particularly troublesome in an otherwise reasonably controlled patient, intra-articular injection of corticosteroid is widely used.

Cytotoxic drugs

Azathioprine, cyclophosphamide and chlorambucil have been the most widely used. Their use as immunosuppressants is discussed in Chapter 12.2.

Comment

No hard and fast rules can be laid down about the use of antirheumatic drugs. The most logical approach is to work through the sequence of first-, second- and third-line drugs moving from one category to the next only when there is convincing clinical evidence of therapeutic failure. Second- and third-line drugs carry a much greater risk of serious toxicity and this must be weighed against their benefits in terms of pain relief and minimisation of joint destruction and deformity. Inflammatory joint disease remains an important and difficult therapeutic challenge.

11.4 DRUGS USED IN GOUT

It is important to distinguish:
  (1) Management of the acute attack,
  (2) Long-term management.

Management of the acute attack

An acute attack of gout is extremely painful and effective anti-inflammatory drugs should be given at once. The drugs used are:
  (1) Non-steroidal anti-inflammatory agents such as phenylbutazone or indomethacin in large doses.
  (2) Colchicine: this drug can still be used in acute gout (orally or intravenously) or in the early months of treatment with allopurinol. Adverse effects, nausea, vomiting, abdominal pain and diarrhoea can be less common with low dose regimens.

Long-term management

As the underlying mechanism in gout involves excess production of uric acid and its deposition in joints and in the kidney, long-term management aims at reducing uric acid in the body in two ways:
  (1) Inhibition of uric acid formation from purines by xanthine oxidase inhibition,
  (2) Promotion of urate excretion in the urine.

Xanthine oxidase inhibition

Allopurinol

Pharmacokinetics

Allopurinol is well absorbed from the gastrointestinal tract and is rapidly cleared from the plasma with a half-life of 2–3 h. It is converted to alloxanthine and this metabolite in turn inhibits the metabolism of the parent drug. Alloxanthine is also a xanthine oxidase inhibitor.

Adverse effects

These are not common. Hypersensitivity reactions which subside on withdrawing the drug consist of a skin rash accompanied by fever, malaise and muscle pain. Rarely, leucopenia or leukocytosis with eosinophilia occur.

Drug interactions

Drugs depending on xanthine oxidase for their metabolic conversion should be given with caution in association with allopurinol. This applies to 6-mercaptopurine and azathioprine. Inhibition of warfarin metabolism may also occur: anticoagulant control should be monitored closely in these circumstances.

Clinical use and dose

Initially 100 mg daily as a single dose, then increasing to about 300 mg daily depending on serum uric acid levels. Colchicine may be given over the first few months to prevent acute gout.

Uricosuric drugs

Probenecid

Probenecid inhibits the transport of organic acids across lipid membranes, including the renal tubule. Whereas this leads to an increase in the plasma concentration of a number of acidic drugs, the uric acid concentration falls because its reabsorption from tubular fluid is inhibited.

Pharmacokinetics

Probenecid is well absorbed from the gastrointestinal tract and peak concentrations are achieved in 2–4 hours. Metabolism and renal excretion result in a half-life of about 9 h; a large proportion of the parent drug is actively secreted by the proximal tubules.

Adverse effects

About 25% of patients experience dyspepsia and this limits its use in peptic ulceration. Hypersensitivity reactions occur occasionally as skin rashes. Drug-induced nephrotic syndrome has been reported.

Drug interactions

The uricosuric effect of probenecid may be inhibited by large doses of salicylates. Aspirin should therefore be avoided in patients receiving probenecid.

Dose

250 mg twice daily initially, increasing to a maximum of 2 g daily over 2–3 weeks, depending on serum uric acid concentrations.

Sulphinpyrazone

Sulphinpyrazone inhibits the tubular reabsorption of uric acid when given in sufficient dose. Like probenecid, it reduces the renal tubular secretion of many other organic acids. This drug also modifies platelet function and is used in the treatment of thrombotic diseases (Chapter 16.5).

Pharmacokinetics

Sulphinpyrazone is well absorbed from the gastrointestinal tract. It is strongly bound (98–99%) to plasma albumin, 90% is excreted unchanged in the urine; 10% is metabolised to the *N-p-*hydroxyphenyl metabolite, itself a potent uricosuric.

Adverse effects

Ten to fifteen per cent of patients receiving sulphinpyrazone develop gastrointestinal symptoms and as a rule it should be avoided in patients with a history of peptic ulceration. Rarely, it causes skin rashes and fever.

Drug interactions

As with probenecid, salicylates inhibit the uricosuric effect of sulphinpyrazone and more than occasional doses of aspirin should be avoided. Decreased excretion of oral hypoglycemic agents may lead to hypoglycaemia and sulphinpyrazone may enhance the effect of warfarin.

Dose

100–200 mg daily, increasing over 2–3 weeks to about 600–800 mg daily, depending on serum uric acid concentrations.

Comment

The modern management of gout aims prophylactically to reduce uric acid formation by xanthine oxidase inhibition with allopurinol and thus prevent arthritis and renal damage. If acute arthritis occurs it should be managed symptomatically with high doses of NSAIDs and allopurinol therapy begun after symptoms subside.

CHAPTER 12

Cytotoxic drugs and immunopharmacology

12.1   CYTOTOXIC DRUGS AND CANCER CHEMOTHERAPY

Aims

Drug therapy in cancer may be employed to:
(1) Eradicate the disease,
(2) Induce a remission,
(3) Control symptoms.

In recent years increasing use has been made of drugs that modify the growth of cells and tissues. Such drugs are indicated in the treatment of cancer, in the control of the immune responses in organ transplantation and in the management of the autoimmune diseases.

Relevant pathophysiology

Chemotherapy or use of drugs in the management of cancer was introduced in the 1890s with non-specific cell poisons. More specific agents became available with the discovery in the 1940s of nitrogen mustard, an alkylating agent, and methotrexate, an antimetabolite. There are now thirty to forty drugs used in the management of a variety of different forms of cancer.

Initially treatment was restricted to patients with leukaemia and lymphomas, but drugs are now used in patients with solid tumours, particularly in childhood.

To obtain maximum therapeutic benefit it is important to define the aims of therapy at the start of treatment as this often dictates the choice, duration and potential adverse effects of the drugs used.

Chemotherapy is only one aspect of cancer management. Although surgery and radiotherapy are of considerable value, increasing use is made of 'combined modality therapy', or the integration of several different approaches to cancer treatment.

Cytotoxic drugs may be used in this context:

(1) After surgery or radiotherapy when tumour mass is minimal (adjuvant chemotherapy),

(2) Together with radiotherapy or surgery as palliative therapy in advanced disease,

(3) Symptomatic treatment where local physical effects of a tumour mass or widespread biochemical effects, e.g. hypercalcaemia, are troublesome.

Principles of drug treatment

Formerly patients were treated with only one cytotoxic drug. Now it is more common to use a combination of two to six drugs given simultaneously, or closely related in time. With a few important exceptions combinations of drugs are more effective than single agents. This is achieved by:

(1) Combining drugs which are active when used alone,

(2) Combining drugs with different mechanisms of actions,

(3) Combining drugs with different toxicities,

(4) Using drugs at doses close to the maximum tolerated levels.

Most drug combinations have been developed empirically. As the number of drugs used increases so the potential toxicity also increases.

Until recently most cytotoxic drugs were used in patients with advanced or metastatic disease. Considerable progress has been made towards curative treatment of some of the childhood cancers and rarer solid tumours. Nevertheless, there are still many forms of cancer which are difficult to treat with chemotherapy. The effectiveness of chemotherapy in a range of malignant tumours is summarised in Table 12.1.

TABLE 12.1 Responses of tumours to cytotoxic drugs

Tumours for which chemotherapy can be curative
Acute lymphoblastic leukaemia in children,
Burkitt's lymphoma,
Choriocarcinoma in women,
Hodgkin's disease,
Wilms' tumour,
Rhabdomyosarcoma in children,
Testicular teratomas

Tumours that are highly sensitive to chemotherapy, resulting in remissions that prolong life
Breast carcinoma,
Chronic lymphocytic leukaemia,
Embryonal sarcoma,
Lymphomas,
Ovarian carcinoma,
Small-cell anaplastic lung carcinoma,
Head and neck tumours,
Acute myeloid leukaemia

Tumours that are sensitive to chemotherapy, where life is sometimes prolonged
Osteogenic sarcoma,
Myeloma,
Soft tissue sarcoma,
Gastric carcinoma,
Bladder tumours,
Prostate carcinoma.

Tumours that are refractory to currently available chemotherapy
Non-small-cell bronchogenic carcinoma,
Carcinoma of the pancreas,
Colorectal carcinoma,
Melanoma

The availability of supportive measures such as platelet and granulocyte transfusions together with therapeutic drug monitoring has allowed much larger and more effective doses of some drugs to be used. High-dose methotrexate treatment is a good example of this. Methotrexate is a potent but reversible inhibitor of the enzyme dihydrofolate reductase, a key enzyme for DNA synthesis. Enzyme inhibition and the toxic effects of methotrexate can be reversed by the subsequent administration of folinic acid. It is possible therefore to give methotrexate at doses of 100–1000 times that used previously, using folinic acid 'rescue' with minimal adverse effects. This method of treatment has been of considerable therapeutic value. In addition to methotrexate, high doses of drugs such as cyclophosphamide, melphelan and 5-fluorouracil have also been tried. When these are employed it is essential that adequate services are available to deal with marrow failure, infection and bleeding. Very high doses of some drugs are used in the hope of eliminating the tumour completely. This technique has been used in association with bone marrow transplantation in the management of leukaemias.

It is common practice to administer cytotoxic drug regimens intermittently. Pulses of drug or drug combination are given at 3–4 weekly intervals, increasing the effectiveness and reducing the toxicity of the combination. In addition to oral or intravenous dosing, cytotoxics may be given:

(1) Intrathecally to achieve effective concentration in the CSF, particularly for drugs that do not readily cross the blood–brain barrier.

(2) Intra-arterially into a limb, the head and neck or the liver.

(3) Intraperitoneally or intrapleurally to increase the local concentration of drug, particularly where rapidly accumulating ascites or pleural effusions present clinical problems.

(4) Topically on to lesions of the skin, vagina or buccal mucosa.

If a drug requires metabolic activation by the liver, e.g. cyclophosphamide or azathioprine, it is of little value to administer it locally, intraperitoneally or intrathecally.

Cytotoxic drugs

Mechanism

Cytotoxic drugs can be classified as follows:

Alkylating agents, including drugs such as nitrogen mustard, cyclophosphamide, chlorambucil and melphelan. These are highly reactive molecules when activated and bind irreversibly to macromolecules in the cell, notably DNA, RNA and other proteins.

Antimetabolites, which are closely related analogues of normal components of intermediary metabolism or DNA synthesis. Methotrexate inhibits folic acid metabolism and the nucleotides (5-fluorouracil, cytosine arabinoside, 6-mercaptopurine) inhibit DNA synthesis.

Natural products. A wide range of drugs has been developed from plants, bacteria, yeasts and fungi. These include:

Mitosis inhibitors: vincristine and vinblastine,

Antibiotics: such as actinomycin D, bleomycin, doxorubicin, and mitomycin.

Others. Several drugs have been identified, often by random synthesis and screening, whose mechanism of action is not fully established but are thought to interact with DNA synthesis or replication. They include nitrosoureas, hydroxyurea, dacarbazine, procarbazine, cis-platinum and hexamethylmelamine.

Steroid hormones and antihormones. These are widely used in cancer management, not only for the treatment of malignant disease, but also for the treatment of symptoms such as anorexia and hypercalcaemia. Drugs used include the glucocorticoid, prednisolone, stilboestrol, in addition to progestogen and the synthetic antihormones tamoxifen and cyproterone acetate.

Cytotoxic drugs may also be classified according to their effect on the cell cycle. Actively dividing cells pass through several phases. Mitosis is followed by a gap or delay (G1) then a synthetic phase (S), a second gap (G2) and mitosis again. Cells may cycle continuously or enter a quiescent phase. Some drugs act at all phases of the cell cycle while others exert their effects specifically at certain of these phases.

Class 1 drugs are non-specific and act on cells whether or not they are actively dividing, e.g. nitrogen mustard. *Class 2* drugs act only at specific phases of the cell cycle, e.g. vincristine, methotrexate, cytosine arabinoside. *Class 3* drugs act on cells in division and at all phases of the cycle, e.g. cyclophosphamide, actinomycin D, nitrosoureas. Most cytotoxic drugs act by interfering with the synthesis and replication of DNA. The molecular basis of action of some widely used agents is shown in Fig. 12.1.

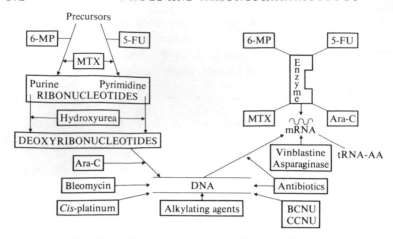

FIG. 12.1   Mechanism of action of cytotoxic drugs

Pharmacokinetics

Pharmacokinetic aspects of cytotoxic drugs include drug specific problems and general problems. Some cytotoxics are metabolised in the liver (methotrexate and cyclophosphamide) while others are excreted unchanged by the kidney (cisplatinum).

Methotrexate is variably absorbed when given by mouth. Plasma level monitoring may help in optimising the dose and in reducing toxicity. Cyclophosphamide is converted to an active metabolite in the liver. Similarly, inactive azathioprine is converted to the antimetabolite 6-mercaptopurine in the liver.

There are further clinical pharmacokinetic problems with cytotoxic drugs:

The problem of the 'third space'. Many patients with cancer have pleural effusions or ascites. Administration of a cytotoxic drug to such a patient may result in the sequestration of the drug into this compartment with slow release back into the circulation. This may aggravate the problem of toxicity.

Sanctuary sites. For many purposes, cancer can be considered to be a systemic disease. It is essential, therefore, that the administered drug reaches all parts of the body. Some of the drugs used do not cross the blood–brain barrier and do not, therefore, act on tumour cells in the brain. Another important sanctuary site appears to be the testes, and tumour relapse may occur there. Clinically, perhaps the most important sanctuary site is the large tumour with a poor blood supply into which the drug cannot adequately penetrate.

Adverse effects

Reactions to chemotherapy are secondary to cell death both in the tumour and in other rapidly dividing cells of bone marrow, gastrointestinal tract, germinal epithelium etc. These can be divided into:

(1) General adverse reactions to chemotherapy,
(2) Specific adverse reactions to individual agents.

General adverse reactions

Nausea and vomiting may be severe and related to the direct actions of cytotoxic drugs on the chemoreceptor trigger sone (Chapter 15.3) or secondary to extensive tissue damage as occurs in radiation sickness. Metoclopramide or phenothiazine antiemetics can be used to control nausea and vomiting.

Alopecia is a common adverse effect of cytotoxic drugs. Hair usually re-grows over months after the drugs are withdrawn.

Hyperuricaemia. Very high levels of plasma uric acid with precipitation of clinical gout or renal failure may complicate treatment of leukaemias and lymphomas. Allopurinol, the xanthine oxidase inhibitor, may be used to prevent gout but care should be taken when azathioprine or mercaptopurine are being given at the same time (see drug interactions below).

Diarrhoea and malabsorption occur as a result of cytotoxic effects on gut mucosal cell turnover.

Bone marrow depression. The bone marrow is particularly sensitive to cytotoxic drugs (Chapter 16.2). Neutropenia or thrombocytopenia are common. They result in an increased risk of infection and haemorrhage respectively.

Opportunistic infections occur as a result of neutropenia and immunosuppressant therapy which interfere with humoral and cell-mediated responses. Unusual infection with fungi and protozoa in addition to more common pathogenic bacteria and viruses occur.

Specific adverse reactions

Specific effects of some of the more widely used cytotoxic drugs are shown in Table 12.2.

TABLE 12.2 Effects of cytotoxic drugs

Drug	Mechanism	Adverse effects	Indications
Cyclophosphamide	Alkylating agent	Haematuria, Cystitis	Haematological malignancy, Solid tumour
Doxorubicin	Antibiotic	Alopecia, Cardiac arrhythmias, Local tissue necrosis	Wide range of haematological and solid tumours
Bleomycin	Antibiotic	Pulmonary fibrosis, Skin rashes	Lymphomas, Testicular teratoma, Squamous cell carcinoma
Methotrexate	Antimetabolite dihydrofolate reductase inhibitor	Marrow suppression, Megaloblastic anaemia	Leukaemia, Choriocarcinoma, Cancers of breast, head and neck
Fluorouracil	Antimetabolite	Marrow suppression	Breast and gastrointestinal cancers
Vincristine	Disrupt micro-tubules	Peripheral neuropathy	Leukaemia, lymphoma and solid tumours
Cisplatinum	Alkylating agent	Renal damage, Deafness and neuropathy	Teratoma and other solid tumours

Drug interactions

With many cytotoxic drugs in use, often in combination, it is not surprising that adverse interactions occur. More important, however, are the interactions noted between cytotoxic drugs, and non-cytotoxic agents.

Methotrexate and salicylates. As methotrexate is highly protein bound it is readily displaced from the binding site by aspirin and other salicylates. This may increase the risk of adverse effects of methotrexate. Other acidic drugs which are highly protein bound may show similar effects.

6-Mercaptopurine and allopurinol. These two drugs are frequently used together. Allopurinol is a competitive inhibitor of xanthine oxidase (Chapter 11.4) and also inhibits the breakdown of 6-mercaptopurine. The dose of 6-mercaptopurine must be reduced by at least 50% or toxicity ensues. Azathioprine, which is metabolised to 6-mercaptopurine, should also be given in lower doses if used with allopurinol.

Procarbazine and alcohol. Hot flushing may occur and patient should be warned of this prior to treatment. Procarbazine is a monoamine oxidase inhibitor and tyramine containing foods should be avoided (Chapter 18.3).

Clinical use and dose

Cytotoxic drugs may be used in a range of malignancies. Leukaemias and lymphomas respond particularly well. Recent reports indicate that some solid tumours may also show a worthwhile improvement. The range of tumours that may respond is shown in Table 12.1 and some of the specific agents and indications are shown in Table 12.2.

Cyclophosphamide: 50–100 mg daily by mouth for immunosuppression, higher doses orally or intravenously as a cytotoxic drug.

Doxorubicin: intravenously into a fast running infusion in doses of up to 450 mg/m^2.

Methotrexate: 50 mg or higher weekly by mouth or higher doses intravenously with plasma concentration monitoring and folinic acid rescue. For patients with leukaemia methotrexate 12.5 mg may be given intrathecally either for treatment of meningitis or prophylaxis.

Vincristine: 1–2 mg intravenously for several weeks together with other drugs for the induction of remission in leukaemias and lymphomas.

Comment

Cytotoxic drugs should be given by physicians who have experience and facilities for managing malignant disease and the problems associated with chemotherapy. Haemorrhage and opportunistic infections secondary to marrow and immune suppression may shorten life rather than prolong it if they are not aggressively managed.

Hormones and antihormones

Oestrogens and progestogens

Surgical removal of endocrine organs such as the ovaries, testes, adrenals and pituitary gland has been used for many years in the treatment of breast and prostatic cancer. Treatment with hormones and antihormones aims to achieve the same effect of changing the hormonal milieu. Hormonal effects are mediated by receptors on the cell surface or within the cells. These receptors, notably oestrogen receptors, can be identified within tumours and allow an accurate prediction of the response to endocrine manipulation in breast cancer. Patients whose breast cancer contains receptors are likely to respond while those without oestrogen receptors are unlikely to respond to oestrogen therapy. Synthetic hormones like stilboestrol and antihormones like tamoxifen, an antioestrogen with very few adverse effects, have replaced ablative surgical procedures. These agents are also used in the management of prostatic cancer.

Aminoglutethimide, which inhibits adrenal steroid synthesis, is increasingly used in the treatment of prostatic and breast cancer.

Progestogens like medroprogesterone are used in uterine, renal and ovarian cancer.

Glucocorticoids

The corticosteroids cortisol, hydrocortisone and prednisolone are used as immunosuppressants in the management of leukaemia and lymphomas. In association with combination chemotherapy they are used in the management of breast cancer. Dexamethasone is used in the management of raised intracranial pressure associated with intracerebral primary or secondary tumours.

Corticosteroids may be useful in the management of complications of malignant disease and hypercalcaemia may be lowered by prednisolone. Appetite stimulation and sense of wellbeing may be improved by corticosteroids or progestogens.

12.2 IMMUNOPHARMACOLOGY

Relevant pathophysiology

The primary function of the immune response is to protect the host from invasion by foreign antigens, in particular pathogenic bacteria and viruses. In addition the immune system rejects tissue grafts from foreign incompatible sources (graft rejection) after transplantation. There are two principal types of immunological response which occur as a result of stimulation of separate populations of lymphocytes.

B-lymphocytes are so called because of their origin from stem cells in the bursa of Fabricius in birds. Their origin in mammals is controversial. They are activated by an antigen to produce specific immunoglobulins or antibodies, *humoral immunity*.

T-lymphocytes derived from thymic stem cells which are activated to produce *cell-mediated immunity* by (1) production of cytotoxic 'killer' cells, and (2) release of lymphokines which in turn modulate macrophage and other cell function. Cell-mediated immunity is particularly directed against viruses, tuberculosis and other intracellular organisms.

'Normal' immune responses may be disturbed in several ways leading to:

Anaphylactic hypersensitivity (Type I). Antigen reacts with antibody (IgE) bound to mast cells and releases mediators: amines, kinins, prostaglandins, etc., e.g. allergic asthma, hay fever, acute anaphylaxis.

Antibody-dependent cytotoxic hypersensitivity (Type 2). Antibodies bind to antigen or cell surfaces and activate cytotoxic responses via complement or other mechanisms:

(1) Organ specific autoimmune diseases: pernicious anaemia, primary myxoedema.

(2) Non-organ specific autoimmune diseases: rheumatoid arthritis, systemic lupus erythematosus.

Immune complex-mediated hypersensitivity (Type 3). Antibody–antigen complex activates both the complement system and platelet aggregation with release of vasoactive mediators locally. Circulating immune complexes may cause the serum sickness syndrome with deposition of immune complexes on the basement membrane of the renal glomerulus and in other tissues.

Cell mediated hypersensitivity (Type 4). T-lymphocytes release lymphokines or are transformed into killer T cells and activate a cell-mediated immune response.

Stimulatory hypersensitivity (Type 5). Antibody directed to a cell surface component like a hormone receptor results in activation of a functional cell, e.g. thyroid stimulation in Graves disease.

Drugs can modify immune responses in several ways.

(1) Suppression of immune responses; used in autoimmune disease, hypersensitivity or organ transplantation.

(2) Suppression of mediator release or reversal of mediator effects; used for example in asthma (Chapter 10.1) and rheumatoid arthritis (Chapter 11.2).

(3) Activation or stimulation of immune responses either via cell-mediated or humoral mechanisms; undergoing evaluation at present.

Drugs that suppress immune responses

Cytotoxic drugs

The antimetabolites **azathioprine** and **methotrexate** and the alkylating agent **cyclophosphamide** are widely used as immunosuppressants at lower doses than used in cancer chemotherapy. These drugs have their effects on actively dividing cells and at low doses appear to have a relatively selective action on lymphocytes. If lymphocytes have been exposed to antigen and stimulated to divide the action of cytotoxic drugs is enhanced.

Azathioprine has a selective effect on T cell-mediated reactions and is widely used in immunosuppression after transplantation and in autoimmune diseases.

Cyclophosphamide also suppresses immune responses but paradoxically enhances cell-mediated hypersensitivity by depletion of suppressor T cells.

Cyclosporin A

This is derived from a fungus. It acts only on actively dividing cells and not on resting cells and has a more selective toxic effect on dividing lymphocytes than other marrow elements. Cyclosporin A is under active assessment as an immunosupressant particularly after transplantation.

Glucocorticoids

Prednisolone and other glucocorticoids have many actions which influence cell-mediated and humoral immune responses (Chapter 13.1). These include effects on:
   (1) Generation of cytotoxic effector cells,
   (2) Lymphocyte recirculation,
   (3) Immunoglobulin production,
   (4) Suppression of macrophage and monocyte functions.
Steroids in high doses are widely used as immunosuppressants but long-term use is associated with a high frequency of adverse effects (Chapter 13.1), and it is preferable to use steroids in lower doses combined with other immunosuppressant therapy (cytotoxic drugs).

Drugs that block mediator release

Drugs that increase intracellular cyclic AMP stabilise the mast cell and prevent degranulation and mediator release. This reduces or attenuates the symptoms of IgE-mediated hypersensitivity reactions.

Beta$_2$-adrenoceptor agonists

Drugs like adrenaline, terbutaline or salbutamol (Chapter 10.1) increase intracellular cyclic AMP, reduce mediator release and improve symptoms.

Theophylline derivatives

These block phosphodiesterase, prevent cyclic AMP breakdown, increase local levels and thus reduce mediator release.

Disodium cromoglycate and ketotifen

These agents stabilise the mast cell membrane and reduce mediator release. The precise mechanism is unknown but may be related to inhibition of phosphodiesterase.

Glucocorticoids

In large doses these have non-specific membrane stabilising properties, which may reduce mediator release and contribute to their overall anti-inflammatory and immunosuppressant activity.

Non-steroidal anti-inflammatory drugs (NSAID)

Indomethacin and related agents block prostaglandin synthesis and interfere with formation of mediator prostaglandins in macrophages and also the leukotrienes. NSAID are useful in the management of some autoimmune diseases, particularly rheumatoid arthritis, but the interference with prostaglandin synthesis may provoke acute asthma in some sensitive individuals.

Drugs that enhance immune responses

Lymphokines: interferon

Lymphokines are released from stimulated sensitised T-lymphocytes. They are soluble substances of molecular weight 20 000–80 000 which modify behaviour of monocytes and macrophages. Although these chemotactic, mitogenic and activating factors have not been used therapeutically, the closely related substance, **interferon**, is currently under evaluation in the treatment of malignant disease, immune deficiency states and viral infections. Interferon inhibits intracellular viral replication and may have cytotoxic effects in some cancers. The therapeutic role of interferon awaits definition following more extensive controlled clinical trials.

Levamisole

This is an antihelminthic which potentiates cell-mediated immunity and is claimed to stimulate immunological responses. The mechanism is not known and the therapeutic role of levamisole is not yet clear. (Chapter 11.3).

Comment

The pharmacological modification of immune mechanisms offers opportunities to attenuate selectively or enhance humoral or cell mediated immunological responses contributing to disease states.

CHAPTER 13

Corticosteroids

13.1   Glucocorticoids

13.2   Mineralocorticoids

CORTICOSTEROIDS

Corticosteroids are usually given for one of three reasons:
1. Suppression of inflammation,
2. Suppression of immune responses,
3. Replacement therapy.

They are hormones normally synthesised from cholesterol by the adrenal cortex and have a wide range of physiological functions. Pharmacologically, they are divided according to the relative potencies of their physiological effects into:
1. Glucocorticoids that principally affect carbohydrate and protein metabolism.
2. Mineralocorticoids that principally affect sodium balance.

Production of the naturally-occurring glucocorticoids, **cortisol** (hydrocortisone) and **cortisone** is stimulated by the release of adrenocorticotropic hormone (ACTH) from the anterior pituitary. Production of the major naturally-occurring mineralocorticoid, **aldosterone**, is controlled by other factors in addition to ACTH, including the activity of the renin–angiotensin system and plasma potassium. Synthetic steroids have largely replaced the natural compounds in therapeutic use as they are usually more potent, may be more specific with regard to mineralocorticoid and glucocorticoid activity and can be given orally. Prednisolone, betamethasone and dexamethasone are widely used as anti-inflammatory and immunosuppressant drugs.

13.1 GLUCOCORTICOIDS (Cortisol and its derivatives)

Pharmacological effects

Inflammatory responses. Irrespective of the injury or the insult, corticosteroids interfere non-specifically with all components of the inflammatory response. This includes reduced capillary dilatation and exudation, inhibition of leucocyte migration and phagocytic activity and reduced fibrin deposition with diminution of subsequent scar formation. (Chapter 11.3).

Immunological response. In high doses lymphocyte mass and immunoglobulin production is reduced as is monocyte and macrophage function. This results in impaired immunological competence (Chapter 12.2).

Carbohydrate and protein metabolism Steroids promote glycogen deposition in the liver and gluconeogenesis, an increase in glucose output by the liver and a decrease in glucose utilisation by peripheral tissues. There is a concomitant increase in protein catabolism with mobilisation of amino acids from peripheral tissues.

Fluid and electrolyte balance. Even glucocorticoids have some mineralocorticoid activity. The principal effect is of enhanced sodium reabsorption from the distal tubule of the kidney. There is an associated increase in the urinary excretion of potassium and hydrogen ions. Oedema is rare but moderate hypertension is not uncommon.

Lipid metabolism. Corticosteroids facilitate fat mobilisation by adrenaline and redistribution of body fat to 'centripetal' areas: face, neck, shoulders.

Mood and behaviour changes. Mild euphoria is quite common with higher doses.

Increase in the number of red cells, platelets and polymorphs but a decrease in the number of eosinophils and lymphocytes.

Increased production of gastric acid and pepsin.

Reduction in bone formation, a decrease in calcium absorption from the intestine and an increase in calcium loss from the kidney. There is also reduced secretion of growth hormone and antagonism of its peripheral effects, so that in children there may be growth retardation.

Adverse effects

The adverse effects of corticosteroids are largely predictable from the wide range of known physiological and pharmacological effects.

Toxicity

Metabolic effects. Patients on high-dose steroid therapy quickly develop a characteristic appearance: a rounded, plethoric face (moon face), deposits of fat over the supraclavicular and cervical areas (buffalo hump), obesity of the trunk with relatively thin limbs, purple striae typically on the thighs and lower abdomen, and a tendency to bruising. Disturbed carbohydrate metabolism leads to hyperglycaemia and glycosuria and rarely proceeds to overt diabetes mellitus. In addition to the loss of protein from skeletal muscle patients also develop muscular weakness, which particularly affects the thighs and upper arms (proximal myopathy).

Fluid retention, which may be associated with hypokalaemic alkalosis and hypertension.

Increased susceptibility to infection.

Osteoporosis, which may cause compression fractures of the vertebral bodies and avascular necrosis of the head of the femur.

Psychosis. A sense of euphoria frequently accompanies high dosage steroid therapy and this may rarely proceed to overt manic psychosis. The increased sense of wellbeing may lead to an improved appetite and contribute to weight gain. Steroids may precipitate a depressive illness.

Cataract. This is a rare complication, usually in children, reflecting prolonged high dosage therapy.

Gastrointestinal symptoms. Dyspepsia frequently accompanies high-dose oral steroid therapy. There is an increased incidence of peptic ulceration and upper gastrointestinal bleeding. Signs of peritonitis which would complicate a perforated peptic ulcer may be masked by the anti-inflammatory effect of steroids.

These predictable and serious adverse effects should lead to particular caution in the use of steroid therapy in patients who have pre-existing peptic ulceration, severe hypertension, congestive cardiac failure and osteoporosis.

Adrenal suppression

The administration of exogenous corticosteroids results in negative feedback to the anterior pituitary with inhibition of ACTH release and the consequent withdrawal of trophic stimulation to the adrenal cortex. In time the adrenal cortex atrophies and when long-term steroid therapy is finally stopped it may be 6–12 months before normal pituitary–adrenal function recovers. Adrenal suppression has two consequences:

(1) Impairment of patient's response to 'stress' (illness, injury, surgery).

(2) The withdrawal of corticosteroid therapy must be slow and supervised.

Short-term therapy (4–6 weeks) can be reduced quickly and stopped abruptly without difficulty. Long-term therapy, particularly with more than 5–7 mg prednisolone daily, or equivalent, carries the risk of adrenal and hypothalamic–pituitary suppression. Withdrawal must be undertaken cautiously and gradually. Assuming that there is no flare-up of the systemic disease for which the steroid therapy was originally prescribed, the daily dose should be reduced by 5 mg of prednisolone, or equivalent every 1–2 weeks until the total daily dose is at the physiological replacement level of 5 mg daily. This dosage should be converted to a single morning administration and at intervals of 2 weeks decrements of 1 mg should be made. The safety of this gradual withdrawal can be monitored by the endogenous plasma cortisol level. In some cases it may prove beneficial to stimulate the adrenal cortex with injections of ACTH, but this is not universally successful and all these patients require supervision and advice for 6 months after steroid withdrawal.

Patients on long-term steroid therapy, and particularly those undergoing steroid withdrawal, require a temporary increase in dose of steroid during periods of stress because of the inability of the hypothalamic–pituitary–adrenal axis to respond normally with an increased production of endogenous corticosteroid: e.g. in times of intercurrent illness. Similarly, patients on steroid therapy who undergo surgery require an increased steroid dosage to enable them to withstand the stress of the operation.

Topical therapy

Topically applied steroids are absorbed through the skin and in the case of very potent drugs, such as clobetasol or betamethasone, adrenal suppression and the toxic effects described above can occur. This usually happens only if recommended doses are exceeded, extensive areas of skin are covered or very prolonged administration is used.

Other effects peculiar to topical application are:

(1) Worsening of local infections. This is particularly important in the eye where ulcers caused by herpes simplex (dendritic ulcers) spread dramatically and dangerously following application of steroids.

(2) Local thinning of the skin. This slowly resolves on stopping steroids, but some permanent damage may remain.

(3) Atrophic striae; these are irreversible.

(4) Increased hair growth.

(5) The use of high doses of beclomethasone by aerosol inhalation can result in hoarseness or candidiasis of the mouth.

Clinical Use and Dose

Hydrocortisone. Used in three different situations:

(1) *Replacement therapy*, when it is given orally in a dose of 20 mg in the morning and 10 mg in the evening.

(2) *Shock and status asthmaticus*, when it is given intravenously up to 500 mg 6 hourly.

(3) *Topical application*: e.g. 1% cream or ointment in eczema; 100 mg doses as enemata or foam in treating ulcerative colitis.

Prednisolone. Used orally in three types of condition:
(1) Inflammatory diseases, e.g. severe rheumatoid arthritis, ulcerative colitis, chronic active hepatitis.
(2) Allergic diseases, e.g. severe asthma, minimal change glomerulonephritis.
(3) Acute lymphoblastic leukaemia and non-Hodgkin lymphoma.

It would be usual to start at 20 mg 8 hourly and reduce the dose according to clinical improvement.

Used topically in ulcerative colitis as a 20 mg enema.

Prednisone. This is metabolised to prednisolone.

Beclomethasone. This is a fluorinated, and therefore polar, steroid which passes poorly across membranes. It is used topically in:
(1) Asthma, when it is given by metered aerosol doses each of 50 μg. Usual daily dose is 100 μg 6–8 hourly. About 20% of this reaches the lungs; the rest is swallowed and destroyed by first-pass metabolism.
(2) Severe eczema, when it is used as 0.025% cream.

Betamethasone.
(1) Cerebral oedema caused by tumours and trauma; given either orally or intramuscularly in doses up to 4 mg 6 hourly. It is ineffective in cerebral oedema resulting from hypoxia.
(2) Severe eczema; given topically as 0.1% cream.

Dexamethasone is used in cerebral oedema.

Triamcinolone
(1) Local inflammation of joints or soft tissue; given by intra-articular injection in doses up to 40 mg depending on joint size.
(2) Severe eczema; given topically as 0.1% cream.

Clobetasol is used topically in severe resistant eczema and discoid lupus erythematosus.

13.2 MINERALOCORTICOIDS

Pharmacological effects

These drugs produce retention of salt and water by the same mechanism as aldosterone on the distal renal tubule. Their main adverse effect is excessive fluid retention and hypertension.

Clinical use and Dose

Fludrocortisone is a fluorinated hydrocortisone with powerful mineralocorticoid activity and very little anti-inflammatory action. It is used in:
  (1) Replacement therapy in doses of 50–200 μg daily.
  (2) Congenital adrenal hyperplasia in doses up to 2 mg/day.
  (3) Idiopathic postural hypotension 100–200 μg each day.

Deoxycortone is used in replacement therapy and is given as an intramuscular injection of 50–100 mg every 2–4 weeks.

Comment

Steroids are powerful drugs. Dramatic improvement in certain severe diseases is matched by equally dramatic ill health due to adverse effects when these drugs are used in mild inflammatory disorders for which they are not indicated. Steroids, therefore, should be used only when other less toxic drugs have failed, or when the severity of the condition justifies aggressive treatment with steroids in high doses. Once control of the clinical state has been achieved, steroid dose should be reduced to the minimum necessary to maintain the desired effect and, if possible, stopped altogether.

CHAPTER 14

Oral contraceptives and other drugs that influence the reproductive system

14.1   ORAL CONTRACEPTIVES

Oral contraceptives have revolutionised the place of women in society. Their efficacy, convenience and overall safety have allowed women to decide if and when they will become pregnant and to plan their domestic and business lives accordingly. They are, however, potent pharmacological agents and the use of oral contraceptives presents an unacceptable risk to women with certain medical or social characteristics.

Composition

The contraceptive pill contains either an oestrogen and progestogen combined, or a progestogen alone. Both of the naturally occurring steroids, oestradiol and progesterone, are ineffective orally because of extensive first-pass metabolism. Thus synthetic compounds are used. At present, the oestrogen is usually ethinyloestradiol or its methoxy derivative, mestranol. The term progestogen is misleading since the progestogens in use as

189

contraceptives are mainly synthetic derivatives of 19-nortestosterone and are often metabolised to oestrogens. Therefore, progestogens can have some androgenic and oestrogenic as well as progestational properties. Those in common use are levonorgestrel, norethisterone and ethynodiol diacetate.

Mechanism

The combined oestrogen and progestogen pill inhibits ovulation. The oestrogen component inhibits the release of FSH while the progestogen prevents LH release. The abrupt withdrawal of progestogen at the end of each dosing period assures a prompt onset of withdrawal bleeding similar to normal menstruation. The progestogen-only pill contains less steroid than the combination tablets and probably works mainly by altering both cervical mucus and endometrium so as to reduce the opportunity for fertilisation and implantation. In addition, ovulation is prevented in about 40% of women.

Pharmacokinetics

The constitutents of contraceptive pills are well absorbed and are eliminated after liver metabolism.

Adverse effects

The most important, but not the most common, adverse reactions involve the cardiovascular system.

Venous thromboembolic disease
(1) The risk attributable to oral contraceptives is:
    (a) Deep leg vein or pulmonary: 8 cases/10 000/year.
    (b) Superficial leg vein: 11 cases/10 000/year.
(2) The risk is increased by:
    (a) Oestrogen content above 50 μg.
    (b) Intercurrent major surgical procedures.
    (c) Blood groups A, B, A B.
(3) The increased risk is confined to those actually taking the pill:
    (a) Develops within first month.
    (b) Remains constant during use.

(c) Returns to normal within one month of stopping.
(4) Pathogenesis:
   (a) Decreased antithrombin III.
   (b) Decreased plasminogen activator in endothelium.

Myocardial infarction and stroke (including subarachnoid haemorrhage).
(1) The risk attributable to oral contraceptive:
   14 cases/10 000/year.
(2) The risk is increased by:
   (a) Age,
   (b) Cigarette smoking,
   (c) Oestrogen *and* progestogen content, but mainly oestrogen.

Age and cigarette smoking multiply, rather than add to, the risks of the oral contraceptives with regard to myocardial infarction and stroke.

Most of the cases are concentrated in women over 35 who smoke.

It is *assumed* that the risk is also enhanced by hypertension, diabetes, obesity and hyperlipoproteinaemia but numbers are too small for statistical analysis.

(3) The risk is not confined to those currently taking the pill, but persists after stopping.
(4) Pathogenesis:
   (a) Acceleration of platelet aggregation.
   (b) Decreased antithrombin III.
   (c) Decreased plasminogen activator.

Hypertension
(1) Blood pressure rises by a small amount in all women on the pill. There is a progressive rise with duration of use. In most cases this increase in pressure is small and of little clinical significance. Less frequently there is a rise to levels for which treatment might ordinarily be considered. The best course of action in these cases is to stop the pill and observe for several months. Rarely, malignant hypertension occurs and should be treated as a medical emergency. Blood pressure should be checked at each clinic visit in women receiving an oral contraceptive.
(2) The oestrogen component is mainly or exclusively responsible.

(3) Blood pressure usually returns to normal 3–6 months after stopping the pill.

Glucose tolerance and lipid metabolism. There is a small decrease in glucose tolerance. Oestrogens increase, and progestogens decrease, high density lipoproteins. The clinical relevance of these observations is unknown.

Additional effects of oral contraceptives frequently include

(1) Irregular bleeding during the first few cycles,

(2) Headaches,

(3) Mood swings.

Less commonly subjects may present with:

(1) Cholestatic jaundice; particularly if a history of jaundice or pruritis in pregnancy,

(2) Increased incidence of gallstones,

(3) Elevation of thyroid binding globulin (does not affect analysis of free T_4),

(4) Precipitation of porphyria.

There is no evidence that oral contraceptives containing low doses of oestrogen either impair lactation or harm a breast-fed infant.

Drug interactions

Oral contraceptive failure with unwanted pregnancy can be precipitated by enzyme induction resulting from co-administration of drugs that induce hepatic microsomal enzymes (Chapter 1.4):

Phenytoin,

Carbamazepine,

Phenobarbitone,

Primidone,

Rifampicin,

Chlordiazepoxide.

Oral contraceptive failure can be precipitated by reduced absorption resulting from altered bowel flora caused by co-administration of broad spectrum antimicrobials. The mechanism depends on the fact that oestrogens undergo conjugation in the liver but hydrolytic enzymes produced by gut bacteria cleave these conjugates and release free hormone, which is then reabsorbed. Broad spectrum antimicrobials prevent this process by altering gut flora and hormone absorption is decreased. When an antibiotic such as ampicillin is prescribed for a woman who is also taking an oral contraceptive she should be advised to use additional contraception during and for 14 days after the course of antibiotic.

Clinical use and dose

No preparation contains more than 50 μg oestrogen.

(1) Combination pill: 1 tablet daily for 21 days starting on day 1 of menstrual cycle and repeating after 7 pill-free days.

(2) Progestogen only pill: continuous administration of 1 tablet daily starting on first day of menstruation.

(3) Intramuscular medroxyprogesterone acetate: this is a long-acting (3 months) progesterone derivative approved for use on a short-term basis in the UK, for example, following rubella immunisation.

The combination oral contraceptive is the most effective form of contraception currently available: the failure rate is around 1/100 woman years. The efficacy of progestogen only pills is somewhat controversial but is probably equal to that of intrauterine devices: i.e. a failure rate of about 2/100 woman years.

Contraindications

These are summarized in Table 14.1.

Patients with diabetes mellitus or mild hypertension should be prescribed a progestogen-only pill.

TABLE 14.1 Contraindications of use of oral contraceptives.

Absolute	Relative
History of thromboembolism	Diabetes
Moderate-severe hypertension	Cigarette smoking
Active liver disease	Mild hypertension
Over 35 *and* cigarette smoker	Age over 35
Porphyria	
Oestrogen dependent tumour	
Impending major surgery	
History of jaundice in pregnancy	
Major haemoglobinopathy	

Ideally, nobody with a relative contra-indication should receive an oestrogen-containing oral contraceptive. However, real life is not ideal and pressure of social circumstances sometimes dictates that the risks of an unwanted pregnancy outweigh those accompanying use of the contraceptive pill; other forms of contraception are less reliable. The presence of two or more *relative* contraindications strengthens the case *against* using an oestrogen-containing contraceptive.

Comment

The widespread use of oral contraceptives is a testament to their popularity. Serious cardiovascular complications are clearly of concern and must be explained to a woman proposing to take the pill. However, they must be explained in the perspective that risk of myocardial infarction and stroke is concentrated largely in older women who smoke and that some, at least, of the morbidity in currently available statistics can still be ascribed to use of now obsolete high dose oestrogen preparations.

Other uses for oestrogens
   (1) Replacement therapy; the most frequent use in this context is control of menopausal symptoms.
   (2) Dysmenorrhoea.
   (3) Dysfunctional uterine bleeding.
   (4) Prostatic carcinoma: these tumours are androgen dependent and administration of oestrogen will decrease androgen production. Remission occurs in 60% of patients with advanced disease.

   Dose   Stilboestrol 1 mg 8 hourly.

   Adverse effects   Nausea, vomiting, fluid retention, heart failure, feminisation.
   (5) Breast carcinoma: in women who are more than 5 years postmenopausal, oestrogens produce a remission in approximately one-third of patients with metastatic disease. The chance of success is higher (as many as two-thirds) if the tumour possesses oestrogen receptors.

   Dose   Stilboestrol 5–15 mg 8 hourly.

Anti-oestrogen therapy

Tamoxifen competes with oestrogen at binding sites on oestrogen dependent breast tumours in premenopausal women. Remission occurs in about 40% (Chapter 12.1).

Dose 10 mg twice daily. Can cause hot flushes and uterine bleeding.

14.2 BROMOCRIPTINE

Mechanism

Dopamine receptor agonist. Prevents the release of prolactin by stimulating dopamine receptors in the pituitary. Increases growth hormone (GH) release in *normal* subjects but suppresses GH release in acromegaly.

Pharmacokinetics

Effective orally and eliminated by liver metabolism followed by biliary excretion.

Adverse effects

Nausea and vomiting may limit dose increases. Postural hypotension can occur. Constipation is common. High doses (> 20 mg/day) can produce a wide range of neuropsychiatric effects including confusion, psychosis, dyskinesias and bizarre choreiform movements.

Clinical use and dose

Hyperprolactinaemia: up to 7.5 mg twice a day.
Post partum suppression of lactation: 2.5 mg twice a day for 2 weeks.
Acromegaly: 5 mg 6 hourly.
Parkinsonism: high doses: up to 100 mg daily (Chapter 19.2).

14.3 CLOMIPHENE

Mechanism

Oestrogen receptor antagonist. Prevents negative feedback of oestrogen at the hypothalamus leading to increased secretion of FSH and LH.

Clinical use and dose

Female subfertility: 50 mg/day for 5 days.
Oligospermia: 12.5 mg/daily (monitor treatment by regular sperm counts).

14.4 TESTOSTERONE

Mechanism

Testosterone is the major male sex hormone and is responsible for secondary sexual characteristics.

Pharmacokinetics

Extensive first-pass metabolism so given either sublingually or by intramuscular injection.

Adverse effects

Virilisation when given to women. Liver tumours when used in high doses. Methyltestosterone causes cholestatic jaundice.

Drug interactions

Oral anticoagulant requirements decreased.

Clinical use

Replacement therapy.
Oestrogen dependent metastases from breast cancer in pre-menopausal women.

14.5 DRUGS ADVERSELY AFFECTING SEXUAL FUNCTION

Several drugs can adversely influence sexual function and the more frequently used are listed in Table 14.2. Remember that patients might not volunteer information about an adverse effect which they consider embarrassing, and which they might not relate to their drug treatment.

TABLE 14.2   Drugs which can adversely influence sexual function.

Drug	Comment
Methyldopa	Impotence; failure of ejaculation; loss of sexual drive
Clonidine	Impotence Difficulty in achieving orgasm (women)
Tricyclic antidepressants	Delayed ejaculation
Phenothiazines	Difficulties in erection and ejaculation
Phenelzine	Delayed ejaculation
Cimetidine	Impaired spermatogenesis Impotence
Isoniazid	Menstrual disturbance
Diuretics	Impotence and reduced libido: mechanism unknown
Guanethidine	Impotence, retrograde ejaculation

CHAPTER 15

Drugs and gastrointestinal disease

15.1   PEPTIC ULCER

Aims

To relieve abdominal pain, nausea and vomiting and to heal ulcers.

Relevant pathophysiology

Peptic ulcers occur in or near the acid-secreting part of the gastrointestinal tract but their cause is unknown. Gastric acid secretion is usually normal in gastric ulcers and is elevated in less than 50% of duodenal ulcers. It is currently assumed that ulcers result from a shift in the balance between the 'aggressive' action of acid and pepsin and the 'defensive' properties of gastric and duodenal mucosa. Treatment aims to redress this balance.

Drugs used in treating peptic ulcer

(1) Antacids,
(2) Histamine H_2-receptor antagonists,
(3) Liquorice derivatives,
(4) Anticholinergic drugs,
(5) Metoclopramide.

Antacids (aluminium hydroxide, magnesium trisilicate)

Mechanism

These drugs elevate gastric pH and therefore reduce the effects of gastric acid. However, the pain relief produced by antacids lasts considerably longer than their effect on gastric acidity.

Pharmacokinetics

Many antacids are available, but it is important to use one which is poorly absorbed. This avoids upsets in acid–base balance with the possibility of phosphate stone formation in the kidney.

Adverse effects

Altered acid–base balance, e.g. sodium bicarbonate. Diarrhoea, e.g. magnesium trisilicate. Constipation, e.g. aluminium salts. Sodium overload if patient is in delicate balance, e.g. magnesium trisilicate.

Drug interactions

There is decreased absorption of digoxin, tetracycline and phenothiazines. Avoid co-administration of antacids with these drugs.

Clinical use and dose

Aluminium hydroxide is usually given as a gel 5–15 ml 6 hourly between meals or when required.
Magnesium trisilicate: 10–20 ml as required or 1–2 tablets as required. These doses produce relief of symptoms. Considerably higher doses probably produce ulcer healing but at the expense of adverse effects, particularly diarrhoea.

H_2-receptor antagonists (cimetidine, ranitidine)

Mechanism

Competitive antagonists at H_2-receptors in gastric mucosa leading to reduction of gastric acid secretion by about 80%.

Pharmacokinetics

Cimetidine and ranitidine are well absorbed and excreted largely unchanged by the kidney.

Adverse effects

Cimetidine is well tolerated in otherwise normal people and only occasionally causes dizziness, muscle pains and rashes. Patients with renal impairment (including the elderly) accumulate the drug and can develop a concentration-related confusional state. Reduced sperm count has been described in patients on cimetidine but the significance of this is uncertain.

Drug interactions

Cimetidine inhibits the metabolism and potentiates the effect of several drugs including propranolol, theophylline and warfarin.

Clinical use and dose

Cimetidine 400 mg twice daily for 4 weeks
Ranitidine 150 mg twice daily for 4 weeks
   Healing rates of 70–80% have been reported for both duodenal and gastric ulcers, but relapse rate is high. Relapse can be greatly reduced by long-term treatment with 400 mg cimetidine at night but the wide-scale acceptance of this approach depends on the long-term safety of these drugs. This remains to be established.
   In addition to peptic ulcer, H_2-receptor antagonists are useful in:
   (1) Reflex oesophagitis.
   (2) Gastrointestinal bleeding in stressful circumstances such as hepatic or renal failure or serious trauma. Cimetidine should be given intravenously at the rate of 50 mg/h. These drugs have *no effect* in bleeding from a focal ulcer.

(3) Zollinger–Ellison syndrome, in which gastric hypersecretion is caused by a gastrin producing pancreatic tumour, can be controlled by cimetidine in doses up to 2 g/day.

Comment

H_2-receptor antagonists have been adopted with enthusiasm by the medical profession. However, this enthusiasm must not obscure the fact that these drugs are not indicated in the treatment of dyspepsia of unknown cause. In particular, the symptoms of an early gastric carcinoma can be masked by these drugs; know what you are treating before you start treating it.

Liquorice derivatives (carbenoxolone, deglycyrrhizinised liquorice)

Carbenoxolone

Mechanism

(1) Increased volume of gastric mucus.
(2) Increased life span of gastric epithelial cells.
(3) Inhibition of pepsin (possibly).

Pharmacokinetics

Well absorbed except in presence of antacids. Highly protein bound. Eliminated by biliary excretion.

Adverse effects

Carbenoxolone displaces aldosterone from protein binding sites and this can lead to sodium retention, oedema, hypertension and even heart failure in susceptible patients. Hypokalaemia occurs in about 40% of patients from secondary hyperaldosteronism.

Drug interactions

Reduces the efficacy of diuretics and antihypertensives. Hypokalaemia may be enhanced if diuretics are also given. Hypokalaemia increases the risk of digoxin toxicity.

Clinical use

Contraindicated in elderly patients and those with renal or hepatic disease or hypertension.

Carbenoxolone is effective in healing gastric ulcer, the dose being 100 mg 8 hourly until healing occurs.

Deglycyrrhizinised liquorice

An attempt was made to overcome the unwanted effects of carbenoxolone by removing glycyrrhizin. The resulting drugs do have less adverse effects but are of doubtful efficacy.

Anticholinergic drugs (propantheline, dicyclomine)

Mechanism

Reduce gastric acid secretion and delay gastric emptying.

Adverse effects

Mainly anticholinergic effects: dry mouth, blurred vision, constipation, urinary retention, tachycardia. In addition, the delayed gastric emptying might even encourage ulcer formation.

Contraindicated in glaucoma, prostatic enlargement, pyloric stenosis, ischaemic heart disease.

Drug interactions

Bioavailability of digoxin is considerably increased because the decrease in gut motility produced by anticholinergic drugs prolongs the time digoxin spends at its site of maximum absorption.

Clinical use

These drugs have been disappointing; the large doses necessary to reduce acid secretion are often associated with troublesome anticholinergic effects. The only value in peptic ulcer treatment is co-administration with an antacid at night to delay emptying of antacid from the stomach.

Metoclopramide

This drug is occasionally used in treating peptic ulcer because of its antispasmodic properties. Gut peristalsis is increased, the pyloric antrum relaxes and gastric emptying is accelerated. There is no effect on gastric secretion.

Comment

In general, a person with mild dyspepsia associated with duodenal ulcer should initially receive an antacid. If this is ineffective or if the dyspepsia is severe then an H_2-receptor antagonist should be used. Benign gastric ulcers should be treated with an H_2-receptor antagonist or carbenoxolone and kept under review until healed.

15.2 DIARRHOEA AND CONSTIPATION

Aims

To eliminate the cause. If this is not possible, or the cause is ill-defined, provide symptomatic relief.

Drugs used in particular types of diarrhoea or constipation

Irritable bowel syndrome

This is a common condition characterised by recurrent abdominal pain, constipation and diarrhoea. Pathophysiology is unknown but bowel spasm appears to be involved and this may be related to psychological stress and/or lack of dietary fibre.

Treatment is initially with high fibre diet, e.g. adding a large spoonful of bran to one meal each day, increasing at weekly intervals as necessary. Drug therapy aims at reducing tone in colonic muscle:

Mebeverine is an antispasmodic which acts relatively selectively on colonic muscle. It is not anticholinergic and has no serious adverse effects. However, results are often disappointing.
Dose: 135 mg every 8 h by mouth.

Peppermint oil is also antispasmodic and has been used successfully in some patients with irritable bowel syndrome.

Benzodiazepines and other minor tranquillisers (Chapter 18) have been used on the assumption that 'stress' or anxiety is an aetiological factor, again with occasional success.

Diverticular disease

This is a common condition in older people. Usually asymptomatic, but if diarrhoea, abdominal pain or rectal bleeding occur a high fibre diet is helpful. This can be supplemented if necessary by various proprietary preparations of bran extract or ispaghula husk which swell with water and increase the bulk of the stool.

Pancreatic insufficiency

Cystic fibrosis is the most common indication for pancreatic enzyme supplements. These preparations contain protease, amylase and lipase to facilitate absorption of protein, starch and fat.

Drugs used in nonspecific diarrhoea and constipation

Diarrhoea

(1) *Drugs that prolong intestinal transit time.*
Codeine phosphate 25 mg (as syrup) given 8 hourly is usually effective and is free of serious adverse effects, but sedation can occur and diverticular disease can be worsened.

Morphine in very low dose as kaolin and morphine mixture is also effective.
Dose: 10 ml 4 hourly. Dependence potential with excessive long-term use.

Diphenoxylate is also an opiate derivative. Usually given together with atropine to discourage excessive use. There is dependence potential and fatal overdose has occurred in children.
Dose is 10 mg initially and then 5 mg 6 hourly.

Loperamide is an anticholinergic drug which can cause dry mouth and dizziness.
Dose: 2 mg 6 or 8 hourly.

(2) *Drugs that increase bulk of intestinal contents.* Various proprietary mixtures containing chalk or kaolin are available.

Comment

A cause of diarrhoea should be sought by clinical history and examination, or microbiological or radiological examination.

Symptomatic treatment is with an opiate analogue and fluids only by mouth in the short term.

Fluid and electrolyte replacement may be necessary in severe cases and in children.

Broad-spectrum antibiotics should not be used in the absence of a bacteriological diagnosis as they may themselves cause severe enterocolitis with diarrhoea.

Constipation

(1) *Drugs that increase bulk.* These are drugs of choice if prolonged or repeated use is likely. Bran or ispaghula husk are suitable.

(2) *Stimulant laxatives.* These drugs stimulate bowel activity in various ways. Their use should be restricted to the short term. Examples include: danthron, senna and bisacodyl. Adverse effects include abdominal pain and diarrhoea. Long-term use can lead to atonic bowel.

(3) *Faecal softeners.* These drugs lubricate the faeces and therefore aid passage along the bowel. Liquid paraffin is the best known, but has several problems. Long-term use can lead to malabsorption of fat soluble vitamins (A, D and K) and to granuloma formation in mesenteric lymph nodes. Aspiration can produce lipoid pneumonia.

Dose: 10 ml as required. Avoid long term use.

(4) *Osmotic laxatives.* These drugs retain water in the bowel and therefore increase the volume of the faeces. Lactulose is the most frequently used. It undergoes bacterial degradation in the colon to unabsorbed organic acids. Indicated in the treatment of hepatic encephalopathy because these organic acids result in conversion of NH_3 to the poorly absorbed NH_4^+.

Comment

Notwithstanding the impressive range of available drugs, constipation can almost always be treated by increasing the amount of dietary fibre in the food: this is effective, safe and inexpensive. If it is desirable for other medical reasons to avoid straining on defaecation then supplementation of diet with a drug to increase bulk might be necessary. Drugs for the relief of constipation are grossly overused particularly by self medication with 'over the counter' preparations (Chapter 22).

15.3   NAUSEA AND VOMITING

Aims

Always try to establish underlying cause and then provide symptomatic relief.

Relevant pathophysiology

Vomiting is controlled by two functionally separate medullary centres: the vomiting centre and the chemoreceptor trigger zone. The trigger zone can be activated by numerous endogenous stimuli and also by drugs such as opiates and cardiac glycosides. This activation leads to stimulation of the vomiting centre which actually controls the act of vomiting mainly via the vagus. The vomiting centre can also be stimulated directly by afferents from the intestinal tract, and also higher cortical centres and the vestibular apparatus.

Anticholinergic drugs (hyoscine, dicyclomine)

Mechanism

Mainly through an anticholinergic effect in the gut with some additional central action. These drugs are particularly useful in vestibular induced vomiting and motion sickness. Ineffective in many systemic diseases or drug induced nausea.

Adverse effects

Anticholinergic: drowsiness, dry mouth, difficulty in micturition, blurred vision.

Teratogenicity. Argument has raged over suggestions that dicyclomine is teratogenic. The case is unproven and, at this time, the drug is still being widely used in pregnancy.

Clinical use

Hyoscine is useful in motion sickness in a dose of 300 or 600 μg. Adverse effects limit its long-term use.

Dicyclomine has fewer adverse effects than hyoscine and, in combination with doxylamine and pyridoxine is given for severe nausea of pregnancy.
Dose: 2 tablets at night, 1 morning and 1 afternoon.

Metoclopramide

Mechanism

It is a dopamine receptor antagonist, but whether this is responsible for antiemetic properties is unclear.

Among various other actions, it improves oesophageal sphincter tone, increases the rate of gastric emptying and speeds transit through the small bowel. It can also block drug-induced vomiting mediated by direct effects on the chemoreceptor triggering zone.

Adverse effects

The most serious, though uncommon, problem is an extrapyramidal dystonic reaction with oculogyric crisis, trismus, torticollis and opisthotonus.

Treat with benztropine 1–2 mg intravenously (Chapter 19).

Drug interactions

The increased emptying of the stomach and bowel transit time increases the absorption of levodopa by delivering the drug more rapidly to its site of absorption in the jejunum and, conversely, decreases absorption of digoxin. May interfere with the therapeutic effects of levodopa by blocking dopamine receptors.

Clinical uses

Vomiting associated with gastrointestinal diseases in general; postoperative vomiting; radiation sickness; some types of drug induced vomiting.
Dose: 10 mg 6–8 hourly. Also available in intravenous and intramuscular formulations.

Phenothiazines

General clinical pharmacology described in Chapter 18.4.

These drugs act on the chemoreceptor trigger zone and, in large doses, also suppress the vomiting centre. Probably work via dopamine receptor blockade.

Phenothiazines are effective against the vomiting of uraemia and neoplastic disease, radiation sickness and drug-induced vomiting. Chlorpromazine in the oral or intramuscular dose of 25–50 mg 8 hourly is usually sufficient. Several other phenothiazines are available, e.g. prochlorperazine 5–25 mg orally or 12.5 mg intramuscular.

15.4   INFLAMMATORY BOWEL DISEASE

Aim

To control symptoms or induce a remission.

Relevant pathophysiology

The causes of ulcerative colitis and Crohn's disease are unknown. However, inflammation is certainly present and there is possibly also a defect in cell-mediated immunity. This has led to the use of drugs that suppress inflammation: steroids, sulphasalazine, and drugs that suppress the immune response: steroids and azathioprine.

Steroids

The clinical pharmacology of these drugs is described in Chapter 13.1.

Steroids are used in ulcerative colitis in two ways:

(1) Topical application as the first measure in an acute attack by prednisolone or hydrocortisone enemas or hydrocortisone foam. Although local application reduces systemic absorption, with prolonged use Cushingoid features and adrenal suppression may occur.

Dose

Prednisolone enemas: 20 mg in 100 ml of fluid once or twice daily.
Hydrocortisone enemas: 100 mg once or twice daily.
Hydrocortisone foam: 100 mg twice daily; this preparation is more acceptable to some patients since it avoids the need to retain fluid in the rectum.

(2) If this approach fails, prednisolone is given orally in a dose of 60 mg each day in divided doses, reducing as symptoms improve. Failure to respond over a period of a few weeks is an indication for surgical intervention.

Systemic steroids as described here are also used in symptomatic exacerbation of Crohn's disease.

Sulphasalazine

Mechanism

This is a poorly absorbed sulphonamide complex with salicylate which is broken down in the gut to sulphapyridine and 5-aminosalicylic acid. These are believed to exert a local anti-inflammatory effect.

Adverse effects

Generally well tolerated. The sulphapyridine is absorbed and can result in the adverse reactions to sulphonamides described in Chapter 9.

Clinical use and dose

Maintenance therapy of both ulcerative colitis and Crohn's disease. The drug should be used indefinitely once remission of the acute phase has been achieved.
Dose: initially 0.5 g twice daily with most patients eventually controlled on 1–2 g twice daily.

Azathioprine

The clinical pharmacology of this drug is described in Chapter 12.1.

Success has been claimed in Crohn's disease but not in ulcerative colitis. However, evidence about the possible superiority of azathioprine over steroids is conflicting.

Comment

The management of inflammatory bowel disease is complex and goes far beyond considerations of specific drug treatment. It involves nursing care, psychological support, dietary measures, correction of fluid and electrolyte imbalance and, in many cases, blood transfusions and surgery.

15.5   MEDICAL TREATMENT OF GALLSTONES

Cholecystectomy is the treatment of choice for symptomatic gallstones. However, if cholesterol stones occur in a person who is considered a poor operative risk, medical treatment might be contemplated if the stones are less than 15 mm diameter.

Relevant pathophysiology

Lithogenic bile is the term used to describe bile whose composition predisposes to the formation of gallstones. The reasons why bile becomes lithogenic are complex but the end result is the formation of bile which is supersaturated with cholesterol. Crystals of cholesterol form and, in combination with other substances, gallstones are formed. Various ways of altering the cholesterol content of bile have been studied, but the most important observation is that the lithogenicity of bile is inversely related to bile acid output. Output is in turn controlled by a negative feedback mechanism and therefore by giving bile acids therapeutically the lithogenicity of bile can be reduced. In practice this does not work with all bile acids and some are too toxic to use but chenodeoxycholic acid and urso-deoxycholic acid have been used with some success.

Chenodeoxycholic acid

15 mg/kg/day for 6 months and response to treatment assessed by cholecystogram. Successful treatment can take over 12 months. Diarrhoea is common as is elevation of aspartate transferase but clinically significant hepatotoxicity is rare.

Ursodeoxycholic acid

8 mg/kg/day again for several months. More recently available then chenodeoxycholic acid and less experience currently available with this drug.

15.6 CHRONIC ACTIVE HEPATITIS

Chronic active hepatitis is one of the few areas in parenchymal liver disease in which there is clear evidence of not only clinical and histological improvement but also prolonged survival following therapeutic intervention. The term includes a spectrum of diseases in which immunological abnormalities play either a primary or a secondary role. The most commonly seen type in Western Countries is the so-called 'lupoid' type in which the patients are young, more commonly female and have positive tests for smooth muscle antibody and antinuclear factor. As with other autoimmune disorders there is evidence of response to both steroids and azathioprine. Chronic active hepatitis with a positive hepatitis B surface antigen is much less responsive to steroids.

Prednisolone alone

This is the regime of choice in most cases. A starting dose of 40 mg prednisolone daily is reduced to 10–15 mg daily maintenance over a period of 6 weeks. Treatment is continued until there is evidence of both histological and biochemical remission which may take several years.

Prednisolone and Azathioprine

In cases where a smaller dose of prednisolone is required, e.g. in diabetic or elderly patients, a combination of 5–7.5 mg prednisolone daily together with 50 mg azathioprine daily can be prescribed.

Comment

Chronic active hepatitis may respond to anti-inflammatory or immunosuppressant therapy and thus diagnosis of this relatively rare form of liver disease should be actively pursued.

CHAPTER 16

Drugs and the blood; coagulation and thrombosis

16.1   ANAEMIA AND HAEMATINIC DEFICIENCIES

Aims

(1) To relieve symptoms,
(2) To correct the underlying disorder,
(3) To replace any deficiencies: iron, vitamin B_{12}, folic acid.

Relevant pathophysiology

The cellular constituents of the blood, the red cells, white cells and platelets, exist as a result of the balance between production and destruction. Blood disorders occur when this balance is disturbed.

Anaemia occurs when the concentration of haemoglobin in the blood falls below the normal for the age and sex of the patient. The lower limits of normal are:
(1) For adult males: 13.0 g/dl,
(2) For adult females: 11.5 g/dl.

The balance between production and destruction may be disturbed by:
(1) Blood loss,
(2) Impaired red cell formation: haematinic deficiency or bone marrow depression.
(3) Increased red cell destruction: haemolysis.

Iron, vitamin B_{12} and folic acid are essential for normal marrow function. Deficiency of any or all of these results in defective red cell synthesis and eventual anaemia. As each of the agents plays a different part in cellular production in the marrow, individual deficiencies are manifested in different ways. Accurate diagnosis is therefore essential before any specific agent is given.

Lack of iron causes *iron deficiency anaemia.*

Lack of vitamin B_{12} or folic acid causes *megaloblastic anaemia.*

If the marrow is deprived of either or both B_{12} and folic acid the blood picture and the marrow look the same, but it is essential to determine which substance is missing. If folic acid is given to a patient who has vitamin B_{12} deficiency neurological damage, subacute combined degeneration of the cord, may be provoked or aggravated.

Iron

As iron is usually absorbed from the gut, a satisfactory response is achieved in most patients when iron salts are given orally. Several ferrous salts are available. There is little to choose between them although they vary greatly in cost. The cheaper salts such as ferrous sulphate should be used unless gastrointestinal adverse effects are severe. Slow-release preparations should be avoided because of unreliable absorption.

The duration of treatment, and its success, depends on the underlying cause of the anaemia. Haemoglobin should rise by approximately 0.1–0.2 g/dl (100–200 mg/100 ml) per day or 1 g/week. The achievement of normal haemoglobin levels should then be followed by a further 6 months treatment in an attempt to replenish iron stores throughout the body.

Adverse effects

Some people cannot tolerate oral iron preparations. The main complaints are nausea, epigastric discomfort, constipation and diarrhoea. A change in the ferrous salt form may help but improvement may be related to a lower content of iron in the alternative preparation.

Dose

Ferrous sulphate, 200 mg three times daily until anaemia is corrected and iron stores are replenished.

Parenteral iron

Oral iron therapy occasionally fails to achieve its objective because of:
  (1) Lack of patient cooperation,
  (2) Severe adverse effects,
  (3) Gastrointestinal malabsorption.
Two parenteral routes are then available:
  (1) Deep intramuscular injection.
  (2) Intravenous infusion.
The total dose of parenteral iron required is calculated for each patient on the basis of body weight and haemoglobin level.

Dose

Iron dextran:
  (1) By deep intramuscular injection, 1 ml on the first day; 2 ml daily or at longer intervals depending on the response.
  (2) By slow intravenous infusion, over a period of 6–8 h. The infusion rate should be increased slowly and the patient observed carefully for signs of a type I hypersensitivity response (Chapter 12.4).
Iron sorbitol: by deep i.m. injection *only*; initially 1.5 mg iron/kg to a maximum of 100 mg per injection.

Vitamin B_{12}

Vitamin B_{12} deficiency demands that vitamin B_{12} should be injected in adequate doses for life. Usually the underlying disease, such as pernicious anaemia, cannot be corrected and the vitamin must therefore be supplied by a route which bypasses the defective absorption mechanism in the gut. Treatment should correct the anaemia and then maintain a normal blood picture. It should arrest, reverse or prevent lesions of the nervous system and replenish depleted stores.

Preparations available are hydroxocobalamin and cyanocobalamin. Both are suitable for intramuscular injection and are equally effective, but hydroxocobalamin is now widely used because of its slower elimination from the body.

A dramatic response often follows within 2–3 days of the start of vitamin B_{12} therapy. Symptoms improve and the haemoglobin concentration rises progressively to normal. An early index of success is a rise in the reticulocyte count which reaches a peak after about 1 week and then gradually declines to normal in the next 2 weeks. Marrow changes reverse rapidly.

Adverse effects

These are rare: probably related to contamination or impurities in the injected solution.

Dose

Hydroxocobalamin 1 mg daily by i.m. injection for 1 week then at 2-monthly intervals for life.

Folic acid

Folic acid deficiency in Western countries is frequently the result of low dietary intake. Less commonly it is the consequence of upper gastrointestinal disease. Pregnancy makes such demands on iron and folic acid stores in the mother that it is routine for iron and folic acid to be prescribed throughout pregnancy.

Dose

5–15 mg daily orally initially, then 5 mg daily for 3–4 months depending on the cause. When combined with iron for prophylactic use in pregnancy, 200–500 μg daily.

Comment

Whatever the type of anaemia, a cause must always be sought. Anaemia is an observation not a diagnosis and there could be an important underlying cause requiring treatment.

16.2 DRUG-INDUCED ANAEMIA

Drug-induced blood loss

Drugs used to relieve pain and inflammation in rheumatoid and osteoarthritis are often associated with chronic, occult blood loss from the gastrointestinal tract. Aspirin ingestion is a well recognised cause of this type of anaemia and all other nonsteroidal anti-inflammatory drugs, e.g. indomethacin, ibuprofen, etc., carry the same risk (Chapter 11.2).

Drug-induced megaloblastic anaemia

Two important mechanisms result in drug-induced megaloblastic anaemia:

(1) Interference with cellular DNA synthesis by cytotoxic drugs such as cytosine arabinoside, 5-fluorouracil or 6-mercaptopurine.

(2) Interference with folate absorption or utilisation by anticonvulsants such as phenytoin and phenobarbitone or the cytotoxic drug methotrexate which inhibits dihydrofolate reductase.

Drug-induced marrow depression

Aplastic anaemia occurs when cellular activity in the bone marrow is suppressed and is usually associated with suppression of white cell and platelet formation (pancytopenia). Drugs causing aplastic anaemia usually incorporate a **benzene ring** with closely attached amino groups. The outcome depends on the dose and the length of exposure, and to less well-defined factors such as the degree of susceptibility, idiosyncracy or hypersensitivity exhibited by an individual.

Certain drugs have a high risk of causing aplastic anaemia. These include cytotoxic drugs and gold salts. In other cases this is a rare idiosyncratic adverse effect: with antimicrobials such as chloramphenicol and the sulphonylureas.

Some drugs have a tendency to suppress white cells, e.g. phenylbutazone, meprobamate and chlorpromazine, while others inhibit platelet production, e.g. gold salts.

Unless the risk is acceptable, as in the treatment of some forms of malignant disease, aplastic anaemia should be prevented at all costs. The risks can be minimised by avoiding known marrow depressants, especially in patients with a history of allergy or idiosyncracy. If the risk is accepted, then every effort should be made to detect early signs and symptoms of bone marrow depression. The patient should be advised that sore throat, fever, malaise, and bruising may be an indication. Regular peripheral blood examination is of limited value. In many circumstances, where the degree of exposure to the causative agent has not been excessive, withdrawal of the agent leads to recovery within 2–3 weeks. Otherwise, intensive therapy is required, including comprehensive antibiotics, transfusion of blood products, administration of androgens and corticosteroids and in extreme cases, bone marrow transplantation.

Drug-induced haemolytic anaemia

A haemolytic anaemia occurs when the rate of red cell destruction is increased and red cells survive for a shorter time than the normal 100–120 days. Many drugs can reduce red cell survival:

(1) Those that inevitably cause haemolytic anaemia (direct toxins).

(2) Those that cause haemolysis because of hereditary defects in red cell metabolism.

(3) Drugs that cause haemolysis because of the development of abnormal immune mechanisms.

Direct toxins

Drugs and chemicals that have powerful oxidant properties are likely to cause haemolysis. Damage by these agents results in fragmentation and irregular contraction of red cells, spherocytosis, basophilic stippling, Heinz bodies, methaemoglobinaemia and sulphaemoglobinaemia. In addition to many domestic and industrial agents haemolytic anaemia may follow:

(1) Phenacetin-containing analgesics, which were popular but have now been withdrawn because they were associated with chronic haemolytic anaemia and renal interstitial damage and papillary necrosis.

(2) Sulphones, used in the treatment of leprosy and sulphonamides, including sulphasalazine.

Interaction with hereditary defects in red cells

Glucose-6-phosphate dehydrogenase deficiency in Negroes and Mediterranean races may give some protection against falciparum malaria, but the red cells in these individuals are abnormally sensitive to oxidising agents resulting in haemolysis.

A large number of compounds may cause this haemolytic reaction, notably:

(1) Antimalarial drugs, e.g. primaquine and pamaquin.

(2) The sulphones used in leprosy, e.g. dapsone and other antibiotics.

Immune mechanisms

Drugs can be associated with two immune haemolytic mechanisms:

Immune haemolytic anaemia. Antibodies may be formed against the drug or its metabolites. Antibodies can only be demonstrated in vitro in the presence of the drug. They may be stimulated by the drug binding directly to red cells, forming a drug-red cell complex (the hapten-cell mechanism, e.g. penicillin and cephalothin), or by the drug itself with subsequent adsorption onto the red cell surface. Activation of complement then causes lysis (immune-complex mechanism, e.g. quinidine, para-aminosalicylic acid and rifampicin).

Autoimmune haemolytic anaemia. Antibodies are formed against the red cells. They can be demonstrated in vitro in the absence of the drug. This not uncommon form of haemolytic anaemia has been most often associated with the antihypertensive drug methyldopa. While at least 15% of patients on methyldopa develop a positive direct antiglobulin test, less than 0.1% develop overt haemolytic anaemia. If the drug is withdrawn, the haemoglobin level recovers but it may take many months for the antiglobulin test to become negative. Other drugs occasionally causing this kind of haemolytic anaemia are levodopa and mefenamic acid.

16.3 DRUG-INDUCED NEUTROPENIA

The most common adverse effect of drugs on the white cell system is a reduction in the number of neutrophils below the lower limit of normal (**neutropenia**). Drugs causing this do so either as part of aplastic anaemia (**pancytopenia**) or as a selective neutropenia which does not involve the red cells or platelets. Drugs causing pancytopenia have been discussed in relation to aplastic anaemia. Several drugs occasionally cause selective neutropenia, e.g. antithyroid drugs, sulphonamides, antimalarials.

Treatment of an established case of neutropenia calls for:

(1) Immediate withdrawal of the offending agent,

(2) The prevention or control of infection in protective isolation,

(3) Granulocyte transfusion if any infection fails to show an early response to antimicrobial therapy.

16.4   DRUG-INDUCED THROMBOCYTOPENIA

Platelets may be reduced in number (**thrombocytopenia**) or function by drugs and chemicals. This may be part of aplastic anaemia or selective thrombocytopenia. The latter is a rare effect of the various drugs including thiazides, sulphonamides and sulphonylureas.

Treatment of an established case includes:

(1) Immediate withdrawal of the offending agent,

(2) Administration of corticosteroids,

(3) Transfusion of platelet concentrate.

Comment

Whenever a disorder of blood cell formation is observed and an adverse drug effect suspected, take a careful drug history and consult reference books describing adverse effects (Appendix I).

16.5   DRUGS USED TO REDUCE CLOTTING AND THROMBOSIS

Relevant pathophysiology

Haemostasis involves a complex series of interactions between the vessel wall, platelets and clotting factors: blood coagulation ultimately depends on the action of thrombin to cause the formation of fibrin from fibrinogen. The reaction cascade is summarised in Fig. 16.1.

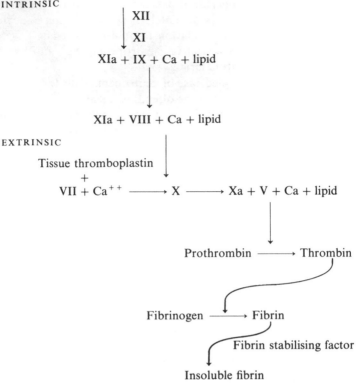

FIG. 16.1   Summary of the coagulation cascade

All coagulation factors (XII, XI . . . etc.) exist in plasma as inactive precursors and most are synthesised in the liver. Vitamin K is required for the production of II, VII, IX and X in the liver from their precursor forms. The clotting mechanism can be modified by interference with the reaction sequence in the following ways:

(1) By potentiating the naturally occurring inhibition of coagulation, particularly at the level of Xa and thrombin: heparin.

(2) Intravascular conversion of fibrinogen to fibrin by an extract of the Malayan pit viper venom (Ancrod): the fibrin is then broken down into soluble products by normal fibrinolytic mechanisms.

(3) Suppression of the synthesis of vitamin K-dependent clotting factors by a vitamin K antagonist: warfarin.

(4) Enhancement of fibrinolysis by streptokinase and urokinase.

Anticoagulant drugs

Heparin

Mechanism

Heparin is a complex polysaccharide which exists naturally in mast cells. Sulphuric acid radicles at physiological pH carry a strong electronegative charge, which exerts the anticoagulant effect. Inhibition of almost every sequence in the clotting mechanism occurs in particular thromboplastin and thrombin generation.

Pharmacokinetics

Heparin is not absorbed from the gastrointestinal tract and must therefore be given parenterally. There is a wide interindividual variability in both kinetics and responses. The *average* half-life is 60–80 min. This means that frequent doses must be given to achieve a sustained effect or heparin should be given by continuous intravenous infusion. High clearance values have been observed in patients with pulmonary emboli, possibly related to increased amounts of anti heparin activity or changes in metabolism and/or excretion. The variability in response precludes attempts to select a dose that achieves a specific effect and dosage adjustments must be made after the anticoagulant effect has been assessed by one or more of the following tests:
(1) Whole blood clotting time,
(2) Thrombin time,
(3) Activated partial thromboplastin time.
Ideally, these should be two or three times control values.

Adverse effects

The principal adverse effect is haemorrhage which is more frequent in elderly patients. The heparin should be stopped. If necessary its effects can be reversed rapidly by giving the positively charged basic protein, protamine. 1 mg protamine neutralises about 100 units of heparin if it is given within 15 min of heparin administration.

Relatively uncommon adverse effects include alopecia, paraesthesiae, thrombocytopenia and urticaria.

Heparin must be used very cautiously, if at all, in patients with peptic ulcer or other conditions likely to cause bleeding.

Drug interactions

Drugs that inhibit platelet function such as aspirin and dipyridamole may provoke bleeding in the presence of heparin.

Clinical use and dose

(1) By intravenous infusion a typical regimen would be: loading dose of 10 000 units followed by 20 000–40 000 units/24 h.

(2) By intermittent intravenous injection: 10 000 units 6 hourly.

(3) By subcutaneous injection into the abdominal wall: 5000 units (mini doses) every 8–12 h are often given prophylactically to reduce the risk of postoperative deep venous thrombosis and fatal pulmonary embolism.

Comment

Anticoagulation is usually started with a combination of heparin and an oral anticoagulant, e.g. warfarin. Heparin is rapidly effective; warfarin takes 2–3 days to achieve full therapeutic effect. Heparin therefore covers this lag period and can then be withdrawn.

Ancrod

Ancrod converts fibrinogen to fibrin which is then broken down by fibrinolysis. There are two adverse effects: (1) haemorrhage, and (2) intravascular obstruction. Haemorrhage can be reversed by Ancrod anti-venom or the administration of reconstituted freeze-dried fibrinogen. The risk of intravascular obstruction can be minimised by giving the drug by *slow* intravenous infusion. The dose is 2 units/kg over 6–12 h by slow intravenous infusion then 2 units/kg 12 hourly by continuing infusion or slow intravenous injection.

Ancrod is an alternative to heparin but is expensive and has few advantages in practice.

Oral anticoagulants: Warfarin

Mechanism

Warfarin and other coumarin anticoagulants decrease the activity of factor VII and then factors II, IX and X. This effect takes 2–3 days to develop as it is the result of suppression of the hepatic synthesis of these factors by antagonism of vitamin K.

Pharmacokinetics

Warfarin is absorbed well by the gastrointestinal tract and is metabolised by the liver. It has a half-life of about 44 h and is given once a day.

The drug used clinically is a racemic mixture of R and S enantiomers. The R isomer is cleared more slowly than the S isomer, which is a more potent anticoagulant. This assumes importance when the isomers are differentially affected by other drugs like phenylbutazone.

There is a direct relationship between plasma concentrations of warfarin and inhibition of the synthesis of vitamin K-dependent clotting factors. It is unusual, however, for warfarin concentrations to be monitored because the therapeutic end point can easily be assessed by:

(1) The one stage prothrombin test, which should be 2.0–3.0 times control values.

(2) The thrombotest, which should have an activity of between 5–15%.

Adverse effects

Bleeding is the main disadvantage of warfarin and other coumarin anticoagulants. It should not occur if control is satisfactory but patients with heart failure, liver disease, who are elderly or malnourished may be particularly sensitive to oral anticoagulants. Minor bleeding (bruising, haematuria, melaena) stops if the drug is temporarily withdrawn. Excessive anticoagulant activity leading to more serious haemorrhage can be reversed by the infusion of fresh frozen plasma or specific factor concentrates.

Because of its long effects (2–3 weeks) vitamin K should be used only if anticoagulation is not to be continued.

Drug interactions

Oral anticoagulants may be involved in serious, life-threatening adverse drug interactions. At one extreme, fatal haemorrhage may occur; at the other, complications from thrombosis may result if anticoagulant activity is lost.

The mechanisms that underlie these adverse drug interactions include:

(1) Induction of hepatic enzyme activity,
(2) Inhibition of hepatic enzyme activity,
(3) Alteration in vitamin K absorption and/or metabolism,
(4) Displacement from plasma protein binding sites.

As one or more of these effects can occur it is not always possible to define the exact mechanism of an interaction, and it is more useful to consider the drugs in common use that diminish or enhance anticoagulant effects (Table 16.1).

The complexity of these drug interactions is typified by phenylbutazone. Initially, when phenylbutazone is prescribed for a patient taking warfarin, there is a transient increase in anticoagulant effect as warfarin is displaced from albumin binding sites. The increase in free warfarin concentration in the plasma is, however, *short lived*, yet the interaction results in a persistent increase in anticoagulant activity. This is because a second, more important mechanism is involved. Phenylbutazone inhibits the metabolism of the more active S isomer of warfarin and enhanced anticoagulation occurs.

TABLE 16.1   Oral anticoagulant interactions

Diminished anticoagulant effect	Enhanced anticoagulant effect
Cholestyramine	Aspirin
Vitamin K	Para-aminosalicylic acid
Barbiturates	Phenylbutazone
Glutethimide	Antibiotics
Griseofulvin	Oxyphenbutazone
Meprobamate	Sulphinpyrazone
Phenytoin	Thyroxine
Chlorpromazine	Clofibrate
Haloperidol	Alcohol
Prothrombin time normalised Thrombotest > 15%	Prothrombin time prolonged Thrombotest < 5%

Clinical use and dose

10 mg daily for 3 days then maintenance depending on the prothrombin time or thrombotest results.

Comment

Oral anticoagulants are employed widely in the prevention and treatment of deep venous thrombosis in the legs and in the prevention of thrombus formation on prosthetic heart valves. There is controversy, however, about the use of these drugs in other thrombotic disorders. It is important to understand that anticoagulants are used to *prevent* further thrombus formation but cannot speed the resolution of existing thrombus. Of the preparations available warfarin and other coumarins, e.g. dicoumarol, are preferable to the indanediones, e.g. phenindione, because they have a lower incidence of adverse effects such as skin rashes, liver and kidney damage and bone marrow depression. Overall, oral anticoagulants are potentially dangerous. Therapy must be carefully controlled. Other drugs, and alcohol, should be avoided and the anticoagulant should be stopped as soon as possible.

Fibrinolytic agents: Streptokinase and urokinase

Mechanism

Unlike anticoagulants, which do not remove thrombus or clots, the fibrinolytic agents streptokinase and urokinase promote the dissolution of intravascular thrombus. The fibrinolytic system activates plasminogen to plasmin which then degrades fibrinogen and fibrin. Streptokinase greatly enhances fibrinolysis and is used in life-threatening venous and arterial thrombosis and pulmonary embolism. Fibrinolytic therapy can be given intravenously for a generalised systemic effect or by local arterial infusion into a coronary artery in myocardial infarction or pulmonary artery in pulmonary thromboembolism. Urokinase, unlike streptokinase, is not antigenic. It is used in patients with obstructed arteriovenous shunts and retinal artery thrombosis.

Adverse effects

The main risk is haemorrhage, which can be reversed with anti-fibrinolytic agents such as epsilon amino caproic acid and tranexamic acid. Streptokinase may cause allergic reactions, fever and skin rashes.

Clinical use and dose

Streptokinase: Intravenous infusion, 250 000–600 000 units over 30 min, then 100 000 units hourly for up to 5 days.
Urokinase: Instillation into arteriovenous shunt, 5000–37 500 i.u. in 2–3 ml sodium chloride.
    Intraocular administration 5000–37 500 i.u. in 2 ml sodium chloride.

Anti-platelet drugs

Relevant pathophysiology

Platelets play a central role in haemostasis and thrombosis. Aggregation of platelets with adherence to vascular endothelium is induced by many endogenous agents, including adenosine diphosphate, thrombin and adrenaline. Thromboxane A_2 (TXA_2) is a cyclic endoperoxide derivative of arachidonic acid formed by cyclo oxygenase and the enzyme thromboxane synthetase. TXA_2 is thus formed in and released by platelets. It is a potent platelet aggregating agent.

Prostacyclin (PGI_2) on the other hand inhibits platelet aggregation. PGI_2 is also formed from endoperoxide intermediates but in vascular endothelial cells. The antagonistic and balancing effects of TXA_2 and PGI_2 by modifying cyclic AMP in platelets control the degree of aggregation and intravascular thrombus formation.

Non-steroidal anti-inflammatory drugs, such as indomethacin, competitively antagonise prostaglandin synthetase or cyclo oxygenases (Chapter 11.2). Indomethacin, however, has little effect on thromboxane synthetase, but aspirin is a relatively selective and long-lasting antagonist of platelet thromboxane synthesis. Aspirin chemically acetylates the enzyme and thus causes irreversible antagonism. As platelets do not contain nuclei they have no DNA and thus cannot synthesise new enzyme. Therefore the block of

TXA_2 formation persists until new platelets derived from marrow megakaryocytes are released into the circulation. The formation of PGI_2 by vascular endothelium recovers rapidly as these nucleated cells can re-synthesise the enzymes responsible for PGI_2 formation.

In addition to the opposing effect on platelet aggregation TXA_2 is a potent vasoconstrictor and PGI_2 a vasodilator. These antagonistic actions on vascular smooth muscle tone may contribute to their role in the pathophysiology of thromboembolic disease.

Principles of drug treatment

While anti-platelet drugs have been widely used in states associated with thrombosis or thromboembolism, in many instances the role of anti-platelet drugs is still controversial and firm conclusions have not yet been drawn from clinical trials. In addition the most appropriate dose and frequency of administration remain to be established.

Cerebrovascular disease

Low dose aspirin with or without dipyridamole is of benefit particularly in transient cerebral ischaemic attacks (TIA) or other symptoms associated with extracerebral, carotid or basilar atheroma and microembolism. Anti-platelet drugs are not of established use in preventing or altering the course of a thrombotic stroke.

Ischaemic heart disease

Several studies have suggested that anti-platelet drugs may help to prevent death or reinfarction in patients who have had a myocardial infarct (secondary prevention). There is no good evidence at present that these drugs have a primary preventive or prophylactic role in angina or ischaemic heart disease. Low dose aspirin with or without dipyridamole or sulphinpyrazone has been reported to improve survival after myocardial infarction.

Prosthetic heart valves and arteriovenous shunts

Anti-platelet drugs are used, alone or in combination with warfarin, to prevent the deposition of microthrombi in patients with prosthetic valves made from artificial materials. Similarly, in patients on haemodialysis with chronic arteriovenous fistulae or after vascular surgery, anti-platelet drugs may prevent platelet aggregation and adherence to damaged endothelium or foreign surfaces.

Aspirin

Mechanism

Aspirin inhibits cyclo oxygenase and thus the formation of prostaglandins and thromboxanes. At high doses (over 900 mg/day) aspirin may influence both thromboxane and prostacyclin synthesis and have little net effect on platelet aggregation. Lower doses (150–300 mg) cause a selective inhibition of thromboxane synthesis which lasts for up to 10 days because of irreversible enzyme inhibition. Recovery is delayed until new platelets are formed and released from the marrow. Aspirin in low doses prolongs the bleeding time for up to 5 days in normal volunteers but does not change platelet survival time if this is reduced by thromboembolic disease.

Adverse effects

Even low dose aspirin may be associated with adverse effects (Chapter 11.2). Gastrointestinal intolerance with or without blood loss is the most important adverse effect. Aspirin should be given as buffered or soluble formulation.

Clinical use and dose

There is still doubt as to the most appropriate dose of aspirin. Soluble aspirin 150 mg daily or 300 mg twice weekly are widely used. Aspirin may be given with dipyridamole as this acts by a different mechanism.

Sulphinpyrazone

This drug was first introduced as a uricosuric agent to increase renal urate clearance. It is also a competitive inhibitor of cyclo oxygenase although selective effects on thromboxane synthesis have not been clearly demonstrated. There are other differences between sulphinpyrazone and aspirin:

(1) Sulphinpyrazone increases platelet survival time when it is reduced in thromboembolic disease.

(2) Sulphinpyrazone reduces platelet adhesion to collagen.

(3) Sulphinpyrazone has some cardiac antiarrhythmic properties.

(4) Gastrointestinal blood loss is unusual after sulphinpyrazone.

Although sulphinpyrazone has been claimed to reduce mortality after myocardial infarction it is not clear which, if any, of the above mechanisms are responsible. Sulphinpyrazone is given as 200 mg four times daily.

Dipyridamole

This drug was introduced as a vasodilator and acts as a phosphodiesterase inhibitor in vascular smooth muscle. This action also leads to increases in platelet cyclic AMP and inhibition of aggregation. Dipyridamole does not appear to have a direct effect on cyclo oxygenase activity or TXA_2 or PGI_2 formation. However, it does restore towards normal the reduced platelet survival time in some thromboembolic diseases.

As a vasodilator, dipyridamole may cause headache, hypotension and flushing in addition to nausea and diarrhoea.

Dipyridamole 100 or 200 mg twice or three times daily can be used either alone or together with aspirin.

Comment

Anti-platelet drugs may have a role in the short-term and long-term management of thromboembolic and thrombotic disease. However, that role, let alone drug dose schedules, is not yet clearly established and may have to await further understanding of the mechanisms of thrombosis. Low doses of aspirin can be given in a convenient simple regimen but may still cause gastrointestinal adverse effects.

CHAPTER 17

Anaesthesia and the relief of pain

17.1 RELEVANT PATHOPHYSIOLOGY

Sensory receptors for pain are found in all tissues of the body. A variety of noxious stimuli (thermal, chemical, mechanical or electrical) cause them to respond and lead to the subjective experience of pain.

(1) The first-order afferent neurones transmitting pain impulses are of two types:

(a) The rapidly conducting (12–30 m.sec^{-1}) small diameter myelinated fibres of the A group (delta).

(b) The slow (0.5–2 m.sec^{-1}) nonmyelinated C fibres. Both rapid and slow conducting fibres enter the substantia gelatinosa of the spinal cord in the dorsal roots.

(2) Second-order neurones carry the pain stimuli to the thalamus in the lateral spinothalamic tracts. Branches from both A and C fibres form synapses with cells in the substantia gelatinosa. The A fibres excite while the C fibres inhibit the substantia gelatinosa cell. The sensitivity of the substantia gelatinosa cells to impulses of the A and C fibres is controlled by descending fibres from higher centres.

(3) From the thalamus, third-order neurones convey pain impulses to the post-central gyri of the cerebral cortex. The thalamus is the main region responsible for the integration of pain input but the cortical area is concerned with the exact and meaningful subjective interpretation of pain.

The transducing qualities of free nerve endings are affected by chemical changes in the immediate vicinity, e.g. changes in the concentrations of potassium or calcium ions, acetylcholine, noradrenaline, 5-hydroxytryptamine, histamine, bradykinin and prostaglandins. Bradykinin and related peptides are formed in extracellular fluid whenever there is tissue damage and account for the vascular and exudative changes of inflammation. Bradykinin sensitises and stimulates nerve endings and causes pain. The analgesic effects of aspirin and other non-steroidal anti-inflammatory drugs result from impaired release of mediator by mechanisms including inhibition of prostaglandin synthesis (Chapter 11.2).

Within the central nervous system, opiate receptors are localised in the substantia gelatinosa and in the limbic areas of the brain. It appears that endogenous opiates released as neurotransmitters from specific opiate containing neurones act at these sites to modify pain sensation. Leucine and methionine enkephalin are pentapeptides which are equipotent with morphine. Beta-endorphin is a 31 amino acid polypeptide formed from beta-lipotropin, a pituitary hormone. It has forty-eight times the analgesic activity of morphine. The discovery of endogenous opiates provides a rational basis for the use and actions of morphine-like drugs. Substance P, an 11 amino acid peptide, may be another transmitter in the pain pathway. It is present in the spinal cord in the central terminals of the C fibres and may be released as the neurotransmitter for the first order neurones.

Principles of drug treatment

From a practical point of view, there are two types of pain,

(1) *Visceral pain* is a dull, poorly localised pain, which is relieved only by potent or narcotic analgesics.

(2) *Somatic pain* is sharply defined and may be relieved by a mild non-narcotic analgesic.

Pain is a valuable symptom of underlying pathology and may be vital in the diagnosis of disease, e.g. in management of the acute abdomen. Unquestioning prescription of an analgesic drug is to be avoided but so also is inadequate administration of relief to a patient in distress.

There is a pronounced placebo effect in the treatment of pain. Thirty per cent of patients in pain experience some relief from a doctor taking an interest in their pain and prescribing *any* drug.

17.2 OPIOID ANALGESICS

Morphine

Mechanism of action

Morphine produces a range of depressant effects by a central action on specific opiate receptors within the central nervous system and in peripheral tissues.

The CNS effects include analgesia, euphoria and sedation; depression of respiration; depression of the vasomotor centre resulting in hypotension; cough suppression; release of antidiuretic hormone; miosis and nausea and vomiting. Peripheral effects include smooth muscle contraction with reduced motility of the gastrointestinal tract; reduced secretion of gastrointestinal tract; biliary spasm; urinary retention; constriction of bronchi partly due to histamine release; vasodilatation and itching.

Pharmacokinetics

Morphine is unreliably absorbed after oral administration because of high *first-pass* metabolism. However, a slow-release oral preparation is now available which results in delayed but sustained therapeutic plasma morphine concentrations. The drug can be given intravenously, intramuscularly or subcutaneously. After intramuscular injection, peak brain concentrations occur between 30 and 45 mins but relatively little of the administered drug crosses the blood–brain barrier.

The major route of elimination is conjugation with glucuronic acid to form morphine-3-monoglucuronide which is excreted in the urine. Only a very small amount of free morphine appears in the urine, bile or faeces. About 90% of the administered dose is eliminated within the first 24 h.

Adverse effects

Many of the adverse effects of morphine represent an extension of its pharmacological effects as a result of relative overdosage. They include:

(1) Respiratory depression, periodic breathing or apnoea,
(2) Hypotension,
(3) Nausea and vomiting,
(4) Constipation,
(5) Tremor,
(6) Urticaria and itch,
(7) Tolerance and addiction to the drug develop readily even when used in clinical practice.

Drug interactions

Morphine delays the absorption of other drugs when they are given orally. In addition, its depressant effects are potentiated by other drugs such as phenothiazines, tricyclic antidepressants and monoamine oxidase inhibitors.

Clinical use and dose

The main therapeutic uses of morphine include
(1) The relief of visceral and traumatic pain,
(2) The relief of anxiety and pain after myocardial infarction or haematemesis,
(3) In acute left ventricular failure (pulmonary oedema) to reduce preload by venodilation (Chapter 7),
(4) Before and during anaesthesia as part of a balanced anaesthetic technique.
(5) In the control of recurrent cough (Chapter 10.4).
(6) Symptomatic control of diarrhoea (Chapter 15.3).

The usual dose for relief of severe pain is 10–15 mg intramuscularly every 4 hrs or as required to relieve pain.

Other opioid analgesics

Many opioid drugs are available and their properties are summarised in Table 17.1.

Papaveretum is a solution containing the pure alkaloids of opium. It has the same uses as morphine.

TABLE 17.1 Comparison of opioid analgesic drugs

	Dose (mg)	Route	Duration of action (h)	Notes
NATURAL OPIATES				
Morphine	10–15	i.m., s.c.	4	
	10–20	Oral as sustained release	8	Slow onset
Papaveretum	20	i.m., s.c.	4	
SEMI-SYNTHETIC				
Diamorphine	5	i.m., s.c.	4	
Oxycodone	10	i.m.	4–6	
	30	Rectal	4–8	Used in chronic pain
Dihydrocodeine	50	i.m., s.c.	4	
	30–60	Oral	4	
SYNTHETIC				
Pethidine	100–150	i.m., s.c.	2–3	
Pentazocine	20–40	i.m., s.c.	4	Agonist–antagonist
Buprenorphine	0.3	i.m., s.c.	8	Partial agonist
	0.3	Sublingual	8	Slow onset
Butorphanol	1–4	i.m.	4	Agonist–antagonist
Dextromoramide	5–8	i.m.	2–3	
	10	Oral	3	Used in chronic pain
Levorphanol	1.5–4.5	Oral/i.m.	4–6	Chronic pain
Dipipanone	10	Oral	5–6	Chronic pain
Methadone	5–10	Oral/i.m.	5–6	Chronic pain

Diamorphine or heroin is more potent and more lipid soluble than morphine. It is metabolised to monoacetylmorphine and then morphine. It is claimed to be less sedative and less emetic than morphine but there is little evidence for this. It is used in acute myocardial infarction and is claimed to cause less marked hypotension than morphine.

Codeine or methylmorphine. Its actions are similar to those of morphine but it is a less potent analgesic. It is used as a cough suppressant, to control diarrhoea and in combination with aspirin or paracetamol as a mild analgesic.

Pethidine is a widely used synthetic narcotic analgesic, which may cause more severe nausea and hypotension than morphine. It is more sedative and has a more rapid onset with a shorter duration of action. Smooth muscle contraction is less prominent and, therefore, it is used in biliary and ureteric colic. Constipation and miosis do not occur to the same extent. Its major metabolite, norpethidine, is active and may accumulate and cause convulsions in patients with renal impairment. The risk of toxicity may be increased in patients taking other drugs which induce hepatic enzymes.

Phenoperidine and fentanyl are opioids used intravenously during anaesthesia. They have a very short duration of action (20–30 min for fentanyl and 30–45 min for phenoperidine). They produce marked respiratory depression.

Partial agonists and opiate antagonists

Buprenorphine is a partial agonist and antagonist at opiate receptors. It is a potent long lasting analgesic drug. Dependence or addiction potential is claimed to be low. Hallucinations do not occur but respiratory depression does and is not reversed by the opiate antagonist naloxone except in very high dose (15 mg or more).

Pentazocine is another drug with agonist–antagonist properties. It produces respiratory depression, hallucinations, less nausea than morphine and is claimed to result in less dependence or addiction. As it increases work load on the heart it is not recommended in patients with myocardial infarction.

Nalorphine is an opiate antagonist, which has a high affinity but low intrinsic activity at the opiate receptor. It does have some agonist activity and may cause analgesia and respiratory depression.

Naloxone is a specific opioid antagonist without agonist activity. It is used to antagonise all of the actions of opioid analgesic drugs. It precipitates withdrawal symptoms if given to addicts or to the neonate born to a mother addicted to narcotics. Naloxone may be given intravenously or intramuscularly in a dose of 0.4–1.2 mg.

When given intravenously, the onset of action occurs within 1–2 min and it lasts 20–30 min. Thus, if it is used to reverse an opioid that has a longer duration of action it should be given repeatedly, by intravenous infusion or intramuscularly.

17.3 LOCAL (REGIONAL) ANAESTHESIA

Transmission of impulses in peripheral nerves is associated with depolarisation of the nerve cell membrane which is the result of an increased membrane permeability to sodium ions. Local anaesthetic agents produce a localised, reversible block to nerve conduction by reducing the permeability of the membrane to sodium. Most of the clinically useful local anaesthetic agents act by displacing calcium from the receptor site on the internal surface of the cell membrane resulting in blockade of the membrane sodium channel. These agents may exist in the charged and uncharged form in solution. The uncharged form diffuses more readily through the neural sheath while the charged form attaches to the receptor. The relative proportion of the charged and uncharged form depends upon the pKa of the drug, the pH of the solution and the pH at the injection site. The smaller the nerve fibre, the more sensitive it is to local anaesthetic block. Thus it is possible to block pain and autonomic fibres and leave propioception, touch and movement.

Local anaesthetics are administered locally and do not rely on the circulation to take them to their site of action. However, uptake into the systemic circulation terminates their effects. The rate of systemic absorption is determined by the:

(1) Pharmacokinetic properties of the drug,
(2) Vascularity of the injection site,
(3) Concentration of the solution used,
(4) Rate of injection.

A vasoconstrictor such as adrenaline, may be used in solution with the local anaesthetic to delay systemic absorption, prolong the local block and limit toxicity.

Local anaesthetics are weak bases with pKa's between 7.5 (mepivacaine) and 8.9 (procaine). Marked changes in the ratio of ionised to un-ionised drug occur with changes in acid–base balance. Thus acidosis favours ionisation and 'trapping' of the drug. They are extensively bound to plasma proteins. Differences in binding between agents may influence the intensity and duration of effect and placental transfer.

Local anaesthetic drugs are of two types:

(1) Esters, e.g. procaine, which are metabolised in the plasma by esterases.

(2) Amides, e.g. lignocaine, which are extensively metabolised in the liver, the clearance being dependent on liver blood flow. With the exception of prilocaine, which is a secondary amine, all the amides in clinical use are tertiary amines. In the liver, N-dealkylation of the tertiary amine produces a more soluble secondary amine which may be active and is in turn dealkylated. Very little of an injected dose of local anaesthetic is excreted unchanged in the urine.

The physiochemical and pharmacokinetic properties of several local anaesthetics are shown in Table 17.2.

Lignocaine

Lignocaine has both local and systemic effects. Local effects include loss of pain and other sensations, vasodilatation and loss of motor power. Systemic effects occur following absorption from the site of local administration or following systemic administration and result from generalised membrane stabilisation. Myocardial excitability is depressed. Adverse effects are due to overdosage and

TABLE 17.2 Comparison of local anaesthetic drugs

Agent	Potency	pKa	$t_{1/2}$ (h)	Onset	Duration
AMIDES					
Lignocaine	1	7.9	1.6	Rapid	Medium
Bupivacaine	0.25	8.1	2.7	Slow	Long
Prilocaine	1	7.9		Slow	Medium
Cinchocaine	0.25			Rapid	Long
Mepivacaine	1	7.6	1.9	Rapid	Medium
Etidocaine	0.5	7.7	2.7	Rapid	Long
ESTERS					
Cocaine	1		*	Slow	Medium
Procaine	2	8.9	*	Slow	Short
Amethocaine	0.25	8.5	*	Slow	Long
Chloroprocaine	3	8.7	*		

* $t_{1/2}$ is very short due to hydrolysis in plasma

include anxiety and excitement progressing to sedation, disorientation, lingular and circumoral anaesthesia, restlessness, twitching, tremors, convulsions and unconsciousness. Coma may be accompanied by apnoea and cardiovascular collapse.

A 1% or 2% solution of lignocaine is used for local infiltration, regional intravenous, or extradural analgesia. The maximum safe dose is 200 mg without adrenaline and 400 mg with adrenaline. The first effects are noted 5–10 mins after administration, and the duration of action is of the order of 2–3 h. Lignocaine is also used in the treatment of ventricular tachyarrhythmias (Chapter 6.2) as it possesses Class I antiarrhythmic activity.

Other local anaesthetics

Prilocaine is equipotent with lignocaine and can be used for all types of local analgesia. It is less toxic than lignocaine because of its greater degree of tissue uptake. Large doses may produce methaemoglobinaemia, which is caused by a metabolite, O-toluidine. It is available in 0.5% and 1% solutions. The maximum dose is 300–400 mg.

Bupivacaine is an amide which is four times as potent as lignocaine and considerably longer lasting. It is available as 0.25% or 0.5% solution and the maximum dose is 100–150 mg.

Cocaine is an ester and is unique in that as well as local anaesthetic properties it is a central nervous system stimulant. It is used clinically for topical analgesia and for its central euphoriant effects in the management of terminal malignant disease often together with opiate analgesics.

Procaine is an ester that has a short duration of action and extremely poor penetration because of its vasodilator properties and its high pKa which makes it ionised at physiological pH.

17.4 GENERAL ANAESTHESIA

Modern anaesthesia is characterised by the so-called balanced technique in which drugs are used specifically to produce analgesia, sleep, muscle relaxation and abolition of reflexes. A single drug is very rarely used to produce surgical anaesthesia.

Intravenous anaesthetic agents

These drugs are used to produce a rapid and pleasant induction of sleep. In almost all cases anaesthesia must be maintained by other agents and thus it is rapidity of onset and not brevity of action that is the most desirable property. The mechanism of action of these agents is not known but it is thought they act in the reticular activating system of the brain. They are all highly lipid soluble agents and cross the blood–brain barrier rapidly. Their rapid onset of action is due to this rapid transfer into the brain and high cerebral blood flow. Action is terminated by distribution of the drugs to less well perfused tissues.

Barbiturates

Thiopentone, the sulphur analogue of pentobarbitone, is the most widely used intravenous anaesthetic. After administration of 4 mg/kg, sleep occurs in one arm–brain circulation time (15–20 sec) but this may be delayed in patients with cardiac disease or shock. Loss of consciousness is pleasant and lasts for 3–5 min. After administration, the initial decay of plasma concentration is very rapid and the half-life of the initial distribution phase is 2.5 min. Elimination is by hepatic metabolism and the terminal half-life is 6.2 h (Table 17.3). Thus the drug is not suitable to be given as repeat injections to maintain anaesthesia because accumulation occurs with a very prolonged duration of action.

The adverse effects of thiopentone include respiratory depression, myocardial depression and vasodilatation resulting in a lowered

TABLE 17.3 Pharmacokinetic comparison of intravenous anaesthetic drugs

Drug	V_D (1/Kg)	Cl (ml/min)	$t_{1/2}$ (h)
Thiopentone	1.6	144	6.2
Methohexitone	1.1	825	1.6
Ketamine	3.3	1296	3.4
Alphaxalone	0.8	1430	0.5
Propanidid			0.2
Etomidate	4.5	740	4.6

V_D: volume of distribution; Cl: clearance; $t_{1/2}$: plasma half-life

arterial pressure. Laryngeal reflexes are not depressed until deep narcosis results and stimulation of the larynx may result in laryngeal spasm. The drug has no analgesic properties.

In the event of an extravascular injection, necrosis and ulceration of the tissues may result because of the alkalinity of the solution. The anaesthetist must take great care that thiopentone is not injected into an artery since this results in precipitation of crystals of the drug with thrombosis of the artery and gangrene of the limb. This complication is less severe when a 2.5% solution of the thiopentone is used instead of the 5% solution. Thiopentone, like all barbiturates, may exacerbate porphyria.

Methohexitone is an oxybarbiturate which is three times as potent as thiopentone. The initial decline in plasma concentrations because of distribution is similar to that seen after thiopentone but the elimination phase is more rapid ($t_{1/2}$ = 97 min). Adverse effects include respiratory depression, muscle twitching and involuntary movements. It is used to induce anaesthesia in outpatients.

Non-barbiturate anaesthetics

Ketamine is a derivative of phencyclidine. It may be administered intravenously or intramuscularly and has both analgesic and anaesthetic properties. Distribution of the drug throughout the body is very rapid and the metabolic half-life is of the order of 2.5 h. When given in large doses, dreams and hallucinations may occur on awakening. This has limited its usefulness. These psychic sequelae may be abolished by benzodiazepines. Other adverse effects include hypertension.

Althesin consists of a mixture of two steroid drugs, alphaxalone and alphadolone, the former being the main constituent. It has a smaller volume of distribution than other anaesthetic agents and a high clearance. Thus its half-life is short (34 min). The popularity of this drug has been limited by hypersensitivity reactions.

Propanidid is a eugenol derivative. It has an extremely short duration of action which is partly due to its rapid hydrolysis by plasma and hepatic cholinesterase. Patients with an inherited abnormality of this enzyme experience a prolonged duration of action. Propanidid depresses the myocardium and lowers arterial pressure. It produces a transient hyperpnoea followed by apnoea.

Etomidate is an imidazole derivative with very short duration of action due to rapid distribution. Metabolised in the liver, it has a half-life of 4.6 h. Injection may be painful and causes muscle twitching with involuntary movements.

Inhalation anaesthetic agents

These agents are used to maintain a state of general anaesthesia after induction. The depth of anaesthesia produced by these drugs is related to the tension or the partial pressure of the agent in the arterial blood. Since the alveolar epithelium of the lung presents virtually no barrier to their diffusion, the alveolar concentration or partial pressure of the drug in the alveoli determines the depth of anaesthesia. This alveolar concentration is influenced by:

(1) The concentration of the drug in the inspired gas,
(2) Alveolar ventilation,
(3) Cardiac output,
(4) The solubility of the drug in blood.

As a general rule, drugs with a low blood–gas solubility such as nitrous oxide, cyclopropane and halothane act rapidly and drugs with a high blood–gas solubility such as ether and trichlorethylene act slowly.

The potency of these agents depends directly on fat solubility. The minimum alveolar concentration (MAC) is the alveolar concentration which produces a state of surgical anaesthesia in 50% of patients.

MAC × lipid:gas solubility coefficient for any agent is constant (200).

Nitrous oxide is a gas at room temperature. It cannot produce surgical anaesthesia when administered alone as its MAC is over 100%. It is used in a concentration of 50–80% to produce analgesia. Prolonged exposure to nitrous oxide may result in bone marrow depression.

Cyclopropane is the only other gaseous anaesthetic agent used. It is explosive and has thus lost popularity.

Halothane is a potent, non-irritant, non-inflammable halogenated hydrocarbon, which is a liquid at room temperature and must be evaporated before use. 80% of an administered dose is excreted by the lungs and the remainder is metabolised by the liver. Hepatic damage very rarely occurs 7–10 days after halothane anaesthesia and may be due to production of a toxic metabolite. Multiple exposures over a short period of time increase the frequency of liver damage.

Halothane depresses respiration and the myocardium. Brady-cardia and arrhythmias may occur if carbon dioxide retention is present. Vasodilatation and hypotension are also seen.

The MAC is 0.75% and halothane is normally given as 1–2% concentration in a mixture of oxygen and nitrous oxide.

Enflurane is a halogenated ether. Its properties are remarkably similar to those of halothane, but it has more respiratory depres-sion and may produce changes in the electroencephalograph simi-lar to epilepsy for a few days after anaesthesia. It is less soluble in blood than halothane and so is more rapidly acting. Its MAC is 1.7% and as the liver metabolises much less enflurane than halo-thane, the risk of hepatitis may be reduced.

17.5 NEUROMUSCULAR BLOCKING DRUGS

When an electrical impulse in a motor nerve reaches the nerve ending it releases acetylcholine at the neuromuscular junction. Acetylcholine acts on nicotinic cholinergic receptors on the muscle membrane resulting in a wave of depolarisation. The acetylcholine is then destroyed rapidly by a specific cholinesterase (Chapter 19.4).

Neuromuscular blocking drugs may interfere with neuro-transmission in one of two ways:

(1) Prolongation of the normal depolarisation, e.g. suxamethon-ium,

(2) Competitive inhibition of acetylcholine at the receptors, e.g. tubocurarine, pancuronium.

These drugs are used during anaesthesia to:

(1) Produce muscle paralysis for abdominal surgery,

(2) Facilitate tracheal intubation and ventilation, of the lungs in cardiothoracic surgery or in intensive therapy,

(3) Prevent fractures during electroconvulsive therapy.

After administration, the anaesthetist must always ventilate the patient's lungs since paralysis is complete. The use of these drugs is an integral part of a balanced anaesthetic technique, but great care must be taken to ensure that the patient is anaesthetised and not just paralysed.

Factors that influence the action of neuromuscular blocking drugs are:

(1) Muscle blood flow (the most important factor). Muscles with high blood flow have the earliest onset and shortest duration of action.

(2) Changes in temperature.

(3) pH.

(4) Potassium concentrations influence the degree of paralysis.

(5) Aminoglycoside antibiotics prolong competitive blockade by reducing acetylcholine release.

(6) Drugs that produce muscle relaxation, e.g. benzodiazepines or halothane, prolong the muscle paralysis.

(7) Renal disease, since all the competitive blockers are excreted unchanged in the kidney to a greater or lesser extent.

(8) Hereditary atypical cholinesterase markedly prolongs the effect of suxamethonium.

Suxamethonium is a very short-acting depolarising neuromuscular blocking drug. A dose of 1 mg/kg produces muscle fasciculations within 1 min followed by complete paralysis for 5–10 min. Respiration must be maintained artificially. The drug is broken down very rapidly by plasma cholinesterase. In patients with the genetically determined abnormality and atypical enzyme, paralysis is prolonged for 6–24 h and artificial ventilation of the lungs must be continued throughout this period. Adverse effects of suxamethonium include bradycardia, muscle pains and raised intraocular pressure.

Tubocurarine is a mono-quaternary alkaloid which produces competitive neuromuscular paralysis. After 15–30 mg intravenously, the paralysis is maximal at 4 min and 50% recovery occurs at 50–60 min. The kidneys are the principal route of elimination with the biliary system an alternative, which becomes more important in renal failure. Neuromuscular blockade may be reversed at the end of surgery by administering an anticholinesterase such as neostigmine. This drug is always given with atropine which prevents the muscarinic effects of acetylcholine and allows the nicotinic effects to be manifest. The adverse effects of tubocurarine include hypotension which is due to histamine release.

Other neuromuscular blockers. Pancuronium, alcuronium and gallamine have a similar action to tubocurarine. Gallamine is less popular because it is completely excreted in the kidney without an alternative route in the bile.

Drugs and psychiatric disease

The last 30 years have seen major changes in psychiatric practice and treatment with the advent of the now familiar range of psycho-tropic drugs and the trend away from custodial care and towards restoring individual patients to a place in the community. The introduction of the phenothiazines in the 1950s brought transform-ation to the lives of many schizophrenics by abolishing trouble-some symptoms and permitting return to more normal behaviour. Next came the antidepressants, a welcome adjunct to the effective but cumbersome and, to some, distasteful electroconvulsive treat-ment. Since the 1960s lithium has been used effectively in acute mania and prophylactically in bipolar affective illness. Last but by no means least, those most widely prescribed of all drugs the pro-liferating array of benzodiazepines, are used for their anxiolytic and sedative effects alone or as adjuncts to other forms of treatment in the whole range of psychiatric illness.

Psychiatric diagnostic categories have a disconcerting tendency

TABLE 18.1 Classification of psychiatric diseases

PSYCHOSES
  (1) Affective
      (a) Manic depressive,
      (b) Depressive.
  (2) Organic
      (a) Acute and chronic brain syndromes,
      (b) Drug-induced.
  (3) Puerperal, postpartum.
  (4) Functional
      (a) Schizophrenia,
      (b) Paranoid states.

NEUROSES
  (1) Anxiety,
  (2) Phobic states,
  (3) Obsessive, compulsive,
  (4) Depressive (reactive depression),
  (5) Hysterical,

LESS commonly behavioural aspects of drug
dependence, alcoholism and personality
disorders may require drug treatment.

---

to merge. Attempts to clarify by reclassification has led to a proliferation of overlapping terminology. In general, where a particular illness does not fall clearly into a diagnostic category, treatment is directed at relief of the predominating symptoms. The scheme above is presented as a working outline of the major categories in which drug treatment is likely to be required (Table 18.1).

Comment

The classification of psychiatric diseases is controversial and complex with frequent overlap. It is important to try to characterise the principal underlying abnormality, as specific drug treatment is available for most of these categories. Misdiagnosis may exacerbate psychiatric symptoms; e.g. sedative benzodiazepines given to a depressed patient may lead to further obtundation of function. Tricyclic antidepressants may precipitate or aggravate psychotic symptoms in a schizophrenic patient.

18.1 MINOR TRANQUILLISERS

Aim

To control symptoms of anxiety without interfering with normal physical or mental function.

Relevant pathophysiology

The experience of anxiety is a universal phenomenon. Excessive anxiety or its physical manifestations, or a perception of excessive anxiety is very common, and it accounts in part for the wide use of anxiolytic drugs or minor tranquillisers (15–20% of the population at any time). At present in Britain as in the United States of America the anxiolytic benzodiazepines are the most widely prescribed group of drugs. Medical practitioners, conditioned to 'treat', find it extremely difficult to acknowledge that a patient's problem lies outside the scope of medical treatment.

Symptoms of anxiety may simulate organic disease and include:
(1) Tachycardia, palpitations, hypertension,
(2) Flushing and sweating,
(3) Nausea, vomiting and diarrhoea,
(4) Urinary frequency,
(5) Dry mouth,
(6) Headache,
(7) Tremor,
(8) Insomnia,
(9) Agitation and apprehension.

The treatment of anxiety states should not be undertaken without a full clinical history, physical examination, and a discussion with the patient of any morbid fears or organic symptoms which underlie the anxiety state. Anxiety is a common accompaniment of physical disease, and not infrequently complicates depression and early schizophrenia.

In certain patients some form of psychotherapy or behaviour therapy may be appropriate.

At present the two principal groups of drugs used in the management of anxiety are the **benzodiazepines** and the **beta-receptor blockers**.

Comment

Anxiety in appropriate circumstances is a normal response. If anxiety symptoms are frequent or persist in a severe form, they may interfere with normal function. Such pathological anxiety is an indication for assessment and possibly drug treatment.

Benzodiazepines

Mechanism

Benzodiazepines have a relatively selective action on the limbic system, cerebral cortex and the reticular formation. There is no good evidence that they act directly by modifying endogenous brain catecholamine or serotonin mechanisms, but benzodiazepines do increase gamma amino butyric acid (GABA) activity. Recently the identification of specific binding sites for benzodiazepines has led to speculation that these 'receptors' are normally present to be activated by an as yet unidentified 'endogenous benzodiazepine', which is lacking in anxiety states.

Benzodiazepines do not have analgesic properties. However, an amnesic action is useful in addition to sedation and is utilised as premedication for minor investigative procedures like gastroscopy and bronchoscopy. Several studies in anxiety have confirmed the anxiolytic efficacy of benzodiazepines and their superiority to barbiturates.

Benzodiazepines currently available range from very short-acting drugs such as flurazepam or temazepam, which are used as hypnotics, to longer-acting agents such as diazepam, chlordiazepoxide, oxazepam, which are most useful as anxiolytics. Variations in pharmacokinetics and metabolism are responsible for these differences.

Pharmacokinetics

Diazepam is rapidly absorbed from the gastrointestinal tract and extensively metabolised by oxidation in the liver. It forms several active metabolites including oxazepam, which is used therapeutically in its own right. The plasma half-life is long (24 h), and its duration of effect even longer, as the active metabolites have half-lives of several days. The half-life may be increased in the elderly, who may also be more sensitive to the drug.

Oxazepam is an active metabolite of diazepam. It is cleared by conjugation in the liver and has a half-life of 10–20 h.

Medazepam is also metabolised in the liver to diazepam. These agents have few clear advantages over diazepam.

Chlordiazepoxide was one of the earlier benzodiazepines. It is still used as an anxiolytic.

Adverse effects

These include:

(1) Drowsiness, agitation, ataxia and 'lightheadedness', especially in the elderly,

(2) Incontinence, nightmares and confusion,

(3) Excessive salivation,

(4) Changes in libido,

(5) Respiratory depression, hypotension,

(6) Impaired alertness with motor and intellectual dysfunction, e.g. driving, operating machinery,

(7) Paradoxical stimulant effects in some violent patients,

(8) Dependence both psychological and physical is now a recognised problem,

(9) Withdrawal can be associated with rebound increased agitation.

(10) Thrombophlebitis may follow intravenous diazepam.

Drug interactions

Benzodiazepines have additive or synergistic effects with other centrally-acting drugs antihistamines, alcohol, barbiturates. This may increase the impairment of motor or intellectual function or worsen respiratory depression. Diazepam and chlorodiazepoxide do not interfere with the metabolism of other drugs and do not interact with warfarin.

Dose

Diazepam: orally, 4–30 mg daily in divided doses titrated to control symptoms and continued only as long as is necessary.

Intramuscularly or slow intravenous injection 10 mg repeated after 4–6 hours if required. Used as a sedative in acutely agitated hospitalised patients or as premedication before minor procedures.

Doses of other anxiolytics are shown in Table 18.2.

TABLE 18.2 Anxiolytic drugs and dose range used

Drug	Group	Daily dose
Diazepam		4– 30 mg
Oxazepam		30–120 mg
Medazepam	Benzodiazepines	10– 30 mg
Chlordiazepoxide		75–100 mg
Lorazepam		1– 10 mg
Meprobamate	Glycerol derivative	1.2–2.4 gm
Propranolol	Beta-blocker	40–160 mg

Comment

Benzodiazepines are effective anxiolytics and relatively safe in overdose. Respiratory depression may occur in patients with chronic respiratory disease or with intravenous dosing. As long-term use may lead to dependence and withdrawal symptoms, they should not be prescribed indiscriminately or for prolonged periods.

Other drug treatment of anxiety

Beta-receptor blockers

Beta-receptor blockers reduce cardiovascular and other beta-receptor mediated effects of increased sympathetic activity. Most experience has been acquired with propranolol, the non-selective beta-blocker. The clinical pharmacology and adverse effects of beta-blockers are discussed in Chapter 8.3. Beta-blockers should be used with caution in patients with a past history of asthma, peripheral vascular disease, cardiac failure or bradyarrhythmias.

Dose

Propranolol 40–160 mg daily in divided doses.

Barbiturates

There is now no place for phenobarbitone or other long-acting barbiturates in the management of anxiety. Benzodiazepines are more effective anxiolytics with less serious consequences of accidental or suicidal overdose. The dependence potential and withdrawal problems with barbiturates are also more serious than with benzodiazepines.

Chlormethiazole

This agent is a minor tranquilliser and sedative used in acute confusional states, and during alcohol or drug withdrawal. It is usually given by continuous intravenous infusion as a 0.8% solution. The dose is titrated to control symptoms without severe respiratory depression. Oral chlormethiazole is used in agitated and elderly patients but has few advantages over benzodiazepines and prolonged use may lead to dependence.

Comment

Anxiety symptoms should only be treated with drugs if they are severe and interfere with the patient's life style, and alternative social or psychotherapy is not possible or appropriate. Treatment should be regularly revised and stopped as soon as possible. Benzodiazepines are effective but beta-blocking drugs may be an alternative with less dependence problems and abuse potential.

18.2 HYPNOTIC DRUGS AND THE TREATMENT OF INSOMNIA

Aim

In the short term to restore normal restful sleep without a residual hangover effect next day and to aid a return to normal sleep without drugs.

Relevant pathophysiology

Insomnia is an interference with the quality or quantity of sleep and is a very common complaint. Insomnia is a subjective symptom and reflects what the patient considers to be the 'normal' length and quality of sleep. Individuals vary in their expectation of sleep. Requirements for sleep may vary and diminish with advancing age. A reduced duration of total sleep time is common in the elderly and may not be pathological. The treatment of sleep disorders requires:

(1) An assessment of the type of sleep disorder.

(2) Assessment of accompanying symptoms of anxiety or depression and their treatment.

(3) Diagnosis and treatment of other physical symptoms interfering with sleep, e.g. pain, nocturnal dyspnoea or urinary frequency.

(4) Consideration of non-pharmacologic strategies, including changes in life style. Simple measures like bathing, exercising, enriched milk drinks or modest alcohol intake at bedtime may help.

Drug treatment should only be offered when the alternatives above have been excluded, and where there is evidence of frequent and marked sleep impairment. Hypnotics should ideally be used for short periods of days or weeks when required, and not given for regular long-term use.

Comment

A successful hypnotic should act rapidly, allow the subject to wake if necessary without severe sedation, and be free from residual hangover effects in the morning. Unfortunately, few of the available agents meet these criteria.

Benzodiazepines

Mechanism

Benzodiazepines exert hypnotic effects by similar mechanisms to their anxiolytic actions but at higher doses. At the peak of drug action in addition to anxiolytic effect, the drugs affect the reticular formation possibly by increasing activity of GABA neurons.

Nitrazepam, flurazepam and temazepam are widely used. They induce sleep within 20–40 minutes of dosing and produce sleep with a reduction in deep sleep (stage 4) and a reduction in rapid eye movement (REM) sleep.

Residual hangover effects with cumulative adverse reactions in chronic dosing may occur with nitrazepam and flurazepam, which have a long half-life and an active metabolite respectively.

TABLE 18.3   Benzodiazepine hypnotic drugs

Drug	Plasma half-life	Active metabolite
Nitrazepam	20+ h	None
Flurazepam	2–4 h	Yes, with long half-life
Temazepam	5–6 h	None

Benzodiazepines have largely replaced barbiturates in the treatment of insomnia. However, they are not without problems. Although they are safer in overdose, benzodiazepines can lead to dependence and should not be prescribed for long periods or without careful evaluation of the individual patient.

Pharmacokinetics

These drugs are rapidly absorbed and are highly un-ionised at plasma pH 7.4. This, together with their lipid solubility, favours fast penetration of the blood–brain barrier. They are metabolised by the liver and elimination half-life differs (Table 18.3). Temazepam appears to have the advantage of a short half-life and no active metabolites. Residual functional impairment is less with temazepam than other benzodiazepines.

Adverse effects

(1) Over sedation especially in the elderly and those taking alcohol, or other sedative agents during the day.

(2) Respiratory depression, particularly in chronic lung disease.

(3) 'Hangover' or residual effects are more common with barbiturates and long-acting benzodiazepines.

(4) Rebound insomnia and vivid dreams may occur after stopping hypnotics and be associated with withdrawal features including fits.

(5) Dependence and abuse potential has been identified. These drugs should rarely be given continuously for long periods of time.

Dose

Temazepam 10–30 mg ⎫
Nitrazepam 5–10 mg ⎬ 30 min before bedtime
Flurazepam 15–30 mg ⎭

Other hypnotic drugs

Barbiturates

Short-acting barbiturates are now obsolete as hypnotics. In addition to the disadvantages already described, barbiturates are more likely than benzodiazepines to interact with other drugs metabolised by the liver, e.g. warfarin, anticonvulsants.

Chloral hydrate and dichloralphenazone

Chloral preparations are cheap and safe. They have been available for over 100 years and are still used in the young and the elderly. Chloral hydrate is a bitter tasting liquid. It is converted by the liver to the active agent trichloroethanol. Dichloralphenazone is a more convenient tablet formulation of chloral and phenazone.

The most common adverse effects are nausea, vomiting and gastric irritation. Dichloralphenazone may interfere with oral anticoagulant control.

Dose

Dichloralphenazone 2–3 tablets 20 min before bedtime.

Comment

Hypnotic drugs should only be used for short periods of time until underlying physical, psychiatric and social factors have been controlled if possible. Short-acting benzodiazepines, such as temazepam, are the treatment of choice, but chloral derivatives may be useful in children and in the elderly.

18.3 ANTIDEPRESSANTS

Aim

To relieve symptoms of depression, restore normal social behaviour and to prevent further episodes.

Relevant pathophysiology

Depression is common in all populations. Pathological feelings of sadness and despair may be associated with physical and emotional withdrawal. Depressive illnesses are a common factor in suicide.

Psychotic depression. Despair with physical symptoms, e.g. anorexia, sleep disturbance, weight loss. Hallucinations and delusions of unworthiness are common. Episodes may be recurrent (unipolar depression) or alternate with mania (bipolar or manic depressive psychosis).

Neurotic depression. Usually follows a precipitating stressful event. Anxiety symptoms are common but hallucinations and delusions are rare.

Drug-induced depression. A range of drugs including sedatives, steroids, opiates and the antihypertensive, methyldopa, may cause depression. The causative drug should be withdrawn if possible.

The neurochemical basis of depression may involve functional underactivity of limbic and forebrain neurons in which noradrenaline or serotonin act as transmitters. The amine hypothesis is supported by biochemical measurement of transmitters and metabolites in vivo in cerebrospinal fluid and in brain tissue at post mortem. There is further support from the therapeutic actions of drugs that modify amine turnover.

Monoamine oxidase inhibitors block the breakdown of intraneuronal noradrenaline and serotonin and may increase transmitter overflow.

Tricyclic antidepressants block neuronal reuptake (uptake 1) of noradrenaline into noradrenergic neurons, or reuptake or serotonin into serotonin neurons. They may alter transmitter levels in the synaptic cleft. The long-term therapeutic effects of the tricyclics, and tetracyclics, probably depend on chronic changes in pre- and post-synaptic receptor sensitivity.

Comment

The diagnosis of depression is complicated by frequent non-specific somatic symptoms, anorexia, malaise, weight loss, constipation.

Conversely, depression often accompanies non-psychiatric physical illness. Suicide by self-poisoning or other means is a serious complication of depression.

Tricyclic antidepressants

Mechanism

This group of drugs includes the closely related agents amitryptiline, nortriptyline, imipramine and desipramine. They competitively block neuronal uptake of noradrenaline and serotonin into nerve endings and in the short term increase transmitter levels in the synaptic cleft. In the long term these agents lead to changes in number and sensitivity of pre- and post-synaptic alpha-adrenoceptors and serotonin receptors in the brain.

All tricyclics have a range of other pharmacological properties that may contribute to their therapeutic actions and adverse effects:

(1) Alpha-receptor blockade,
(2) Anticholinergic effects,
(3) Non-specific sedative actions.

The therapeutic response to tricyclics develops over 2–3 weeks. Suicide by overdose of antidepressant is not uncommon during this lag period.

Recent reports suggest that long-term tricyclic treatment is superior to placebo in reducing the frequency of recurrent depressive symptoms. Amitriptyline, which has more sedative properties, may be useful in agitated depression or where insomnia is troublesome. Imipramine, with less sedative properties, is indicated in those who have marked motor retardation.

Pharmacokinetics

Tricyclics are extensively metabolised by the liver. The half-life of amitriptyline is >24 hours and the formation of metabolites with antidepressant activity further extends the duration of drug activity. Once-daily dosing, ideally at night, is indicated for most tricyclics.

Hepatic metabolism of tricyclics is determined by genetic and environmental factors. There are wide differences in plasma level

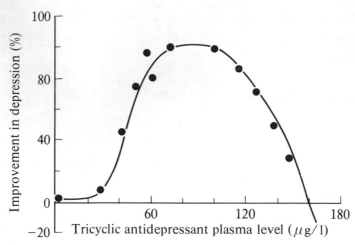

FIG. 18.1 Relationship between drug plasma level and effect in tricyclic antidepressants.

when the same dose is given to a group of individuals. Thus the dose of tricyclic should be individually titrated with therapeutic response or adverse effects as end points.

Studies with tricyclics have shown an unusual relationship between drug plasma level and effect (Fig. 18.1). At low drug levels and also at high drug levels there is little effect, while optimal effect is seen within a very *narrow concentration range* (50–150 ng/ml) *or therapeutic window*. This has led some to propose routine drug level monitoring as a guide to antidepressant therapy.

Adverse effects

(1) Sedation and confusional states, especially amitriptyline,

(2) Anticholinergic effects, e.g. dry mouth, constipation, urinary symptoms, and precipitation of glaucoma,

(3) Postural hypotension, especially in the very young and old,

(4) Cardiac tachyarrhythmias (seen in overdose). May occur more frequently in patients treated with long-term tricyclics,

(5) Self-poisoning by tricyclic overdose is common and its management discussed further in Chapter 21.2.

(6) Fits may occur on withdrawal of tricyclics.

Clinical use and dose

Imipramine ⎱ 25–75 mg orally, titrated to 100–200 mg daily as a
Amitriptyline ⎰ single bedtime dose.

They may also be useful in nocturnal enuresis and hyperactivity syndrome in childhood.

Comment

Tricyclic antidepressants are widely used in the treatment of acute depression and may reduce the frequency of recurrent episodes. There is a delay of 14–21 days before the therapeutic effect appears. The dose should be individually determined. Plasma level monitoring may help in optimising the response in poor responders.

Tetracyclic antidepressants

Mianserin is an example of this group. Its mechanism of action is not clear, but it may block neuronal uptake and with long-term use modify serotonin and/or adrenergic receptors.

These agents have similar therapeutic activity to tricyclics and also a lag in response of 1–2 weeks.

Advantages over tricyclics appear to be the lower frequency of anticholinergic and cardiac side effects, particularly in the elderly.

Dose

Mianserin 30–60 mg daily at bedtime increasing if necessary and if tolerated to 200 mg daily.

Monoamine oxidase inhibitors

Mechanism

Phenelzine, tranylcypromine and iproniazid are non-competitive irreversible antagonists of monoamine oxidase (MAO). The enzyme is blocked not only in brain monoamine neurons, but also in peripheral neurons, enterocytes in the gut wall and platelets. Inhibition of MAO leads to increases in serotonin, noradrenaline and dopamine in the brain.

The problems with MAO inhibitors result from widespread enzyme inhibition. These drugs are rarely used now. Indications are therapeutic failure with tricyclic or tetracyclic drugs, hypochondriasis, phobic states and atypical depression. When used the response may be delayed for 2–3 weeks. Recovery of MAO is slow (2–3 weeks) after the drug is stopped as it requires synthesis of new MAO enzyme.

Adverse effects

(1) Postural hypotension,
(2) Headache,
(3) Anticholinergic side effects,
(4) Drug-induced liver damage (phenelzine and isocarboxazid),
(5) Hypertensive crisis.

The most important adverse effect is hypertensive crisis following amine containing foods, beverages or drugs. Inhibition in the gut wall of MAO allows absorption of tyramine and other sympathomimetic substances in food or drink. These are usually metabolised to inactive products by MAO during absorption. The amines are taken up from the circulation by peripheral sympathetic nerve endings. They displace endogenous noradrenaline from storage sites (indirect sympathomimetic action) and this leads to hypertension, tachycardia and headache.

Severe paroxysmal hypertension may cause a cerebrovascular accident. Foods rich in tyramine particularly cheese, meat, yeast extract, red wine, etc. should be avoided.

Comment

The dangers of hypertension, the limitations on food intake and the availability of tricyclics as alternatives have greatly reduced the role of monoamine oxidase inhibitors in depression.

18.4 NEUROLEPTIC DRUGS (ANTIPSYCHOTICS, MAJOR TRANQUILLISERS)

Aim

To reverse cognitive, affective and motor disturbances and to restore the patient to as near normal a life in society as possible.

Relevant pathophysiology

The neuroleptics, major tranquillisers, are used primarily in the functional psychoses in which they produce a wide range of symptom relief with diminution of delusions, hallucinations, social inappropriateness and anxiety. Studies have shown that up to 90% of patients diagnosed as schizophrenic are helped by neuroleptic drugs.

Presenting symptoms include blunted or inappropriate affect, thought disorder, hallucinations, delusions, impaired emotional response and occasionally bizarre motor or posture disturbance. Onset may be insidious as in schizophrenia or acute, as in the schizophreniform psychoses. In the former a progressive deterioration may follow, while the latter characteristically remits with preservation of personality function. In paranoid states there is a well developed delusional component in an otherwise intact personality with coherent thinking. Drug-induced psychosis may be clinically indistinguishable from the functional psychoses and in addition to withdrawing the offending drug, the symptoms should be treated with neuroleptics if they are severe. The neurochemical basis of schizophrenia and other psychoses has been extensively investigated. The precipitation of psychoses by levodopa and bromocriptine, which respectively stimulate dopamine receptors indirectly or directly, and amphetamine which displaces dopamine from storage sites, suggests that increased brain dopamine activity may contribute to psychotic thought disorder. This hypothesis is further supported by the observation that all the active antipsychotic drugs share a dopamine receptor blocking action. However, functional overactivity of a mesolimbic dopaminergic pathway is unlikely to be the entire abnormality.

Phenothiazines

Mechanism

Neuroleptic antipsychotics all act as competitive antagonists of dopamine receptors in the central nervous system and compete for dopamine-binding sites in vitro.

This series of drugs shows a range of other pharmacological properties which may be of importance in determining the profile of adverse effects for an individual drug.

(1) Anticholinergic activity is considerable with thioridazine and much less with fluphenazine.

(2) Alpha-receptor blockade is prominent with chlorpromazine and thioridazine and less with fluphenazine.

(3) Sedation occurs with chlorpromazine and thioridazine.

Chlorpromazine, thioridazine and trifluoperazine are among the agents used for long-term oral therapy. Fluphenazine in depot preparations may be given by intramuscular injection.

Extrapyramidal (Parkinsonian) adverse effects often occur and may require to be controlled by co-administration of anticholinergic drugs such as benzhexol, orphenadrine, benztropine (Chapter 19.2).

Pharmacokinetics

Chlorpromazine is absorbed orally and metabolised by the liver to many active and inactive metabolites. It has a plasma half-life of over 16 h which, together with the long-lived active metabolites, makes once daily dosing practical. No clear cut therapeutic range can be defined because of the presence of unquantitated active metabolites and a wide range of inter-individual responses in patients. Plasma or urine drug levels are only of help in assessing compliance.

Adverse reactions

Dose related from known pharmacological properties

(1) Dopamine receptor blockade, e.g. extrapyramidal dystonia in the young, Parkinsonism in the elderly.

(2) Increased prolactin, e.g. galactorrhoea, infertility, and impotence.

(3) Anticholinergic effects, e.g. blurred vision, constipation, urinary hesitancy, dry mouth, tachycardia or arrhythmias.

(4) Alpha-receptor blockade, e.g. postural hypotension.

(5) Tardive dyskinesia; these involuntary choreoathetoid movements, unlike dystonia, may persist even after withdrawal of the neuroleptic drug. They may be aggravated by anticholinergic drugs and treatment is generally unsatisfactory. Benzodiazepines, diazepam and clonazepam may be helpful.

(6) Other adverse effects include:
(a) Sedation,
(b) Confusion,
(c) Nightmares,
(d) Insomnia.

Hypersensitivity reactions not related to dose. Cholestatic jaundice with portal infiltration occurs in 2–4% of patients, usually early in treatment. It presents the biochemical features of cholestasis and resolves slowly on drug withdrawal. Agranulocytosis occurs rarely. Skin rashes including photosensitivity dermatitis and urticaria may be seen.

Clinical use and dose

Chlorpromazine: orally 100 mg daily, increasing up to 1 g gradually if required.

Chlorpromazine intramuscular injection, 25–50 mg 6–8 hourly as required to control acute symptoms.

Neuroleptics administered in lower doses are used in nausea and vomiting (Chapter 15.3) hiccough, vertigo and labyrinthine disturbances, and during drug withdrawal reactions.

In acute attacks of mania, phenothiazines in high doses are used. They are widely used as premedication in anaesthesia (Chapter 17.4).

Fluphenazine

Another phenothiazine derivative. As the decanoate or enanthate ester it can be given as a depot by intramuscular injection at intervals of 14–40 days. Outpatient treatment of schizophrenia is aided by use of these depot formulations and the ensuing improvement in compliance. Patients with psychoses are notoriously 'poor compliers' with medical instructions if not under close supervision.

Adverse effects of fluphenazine are similar to those of chlorpromazine but sedation and anticholinergic adverse effects are less common. Extrapyramidal adverse effects are correspondingly more common, particularly dystonia and akathisia or restlessness. Liver and bone marrow toxicity and skin rashes have been reported as with most other phenothiazines.

Dose

Fluphenazine decanoate 25 mg by injection into the gluteal muscles every 15–40 days. A test dose (12.5 mg) should be given when treatment is begun, to assess possible extrapyramidal reactions.

Non-phenothiazine neuroleptics

Newer antipsychotic agents have been introduced, which are not phenothiazine derivatives but share the property of dopamine receptor blockade:
(1) Haloperidol, which is a butyrophenone,
(2) Pimozide, which is a diphenylbutylperidine,
(3) Flupenthixol, which is a thioxanthene.
These agents are less sedating than chlorpromazine and thus useful in withdrawn psychotic patients. Extrapyramidal reactions occur with all of these, but are particularly troublesome with flupenthixol and haloperidol. Pimozide is said to cause fewer dystonic reactions especially at low doses. Flupenthixol as the decanoate can be given by intermittent (2–4 weeks) intramuscular injection.

Comment

Neuroleptic antipsychotic drugs have a major place in the management of functional psychoses. The dose should be individually determined from response and adverse effects. Depot intramuscular preparations may be useful for long-term outpatient management. Adverse effects are common and may be disabling or even dangerous. Patients on long-term antipsychotic medication should be under close medical supervision.

Neuroleptics should *not* be used in the management of simple anxiety as an alternative to anxiolytics or minor tranquillisers.

18.5 LITHIUM

Relevant pathophysiology

Mania and hypomania describe an extreme of behaviour characterised by a pathologically elevated mood. It may present on its own or may be part of a manicdepressive (bipolar depression) syndrome. Mania is characterised by cheerfulness with motor overactivity, non-stop talk, flight of ideas, grandiosity, and a progressive lack of contact with reality.

Treatment of an acute manic episode includes sedation with phenothiazines or other major tranquillisers, together with general supportive measures. Specific therapy with lithium salts is used both in the acute attack and for prophylaxis between attacks.

Lithium carbonate

Mechanism

The monovalent cation lithium, given as the carbonate salt, modifies the affect in mania. The mechanism of action of lithium is not clear. It appears to substitute for the cations sodium and potassium in cellular transport processes. It has effects on release of monoamine neurotransmitters and alters intracellular and extracellular ion concentrations and fluxes across excitable membranes. Lithium may take several days to achieve its effect.

Pharmacokinetics

Lithium is rapidly and completely absorbed after oral dosing. It is not metabolised and is excreted unchanged by the kidney with a half-life of 20 h. Lithium is distributed in total body water, slowly enters cells and reaches steady state levels after dosing for 5 days. There is a very narrow therapeutic range for lithium (0.6–1.2 mmol/l), with severe adverse effects occurring at higher levels. Monitoring of drug levels in plasma is essential for optimal control of therapy (Chapter 5.1). Changes in renal function are the most important factors modifying elimination and thus plasma levels. Lithium clearance is 0.2 times creatinine clearance, and the dose must be modified in the presence of renal impairment and in the elderly. The sodium and potassium status of the patient also influences lithium levels and response. Thus dehydration, salt depletion or diuretic therapy modifies plasma drug concentration.

Adverse effects

These are more common and severe when the plasma lithium level exceeds 1.2 mmol/l or in the presence of salt depletion or diuretic therapy:

(1) Nausea and vomiting,
(2) Drowsiness, confusion and fits,
(3) Ataxia, nystagmus and dysarthria,
(4) Hypothyroidism, by interference with iodination,
(5) Oedema and weight gain,
(6) Nephrogenic diabetes insipidus.

Dose

Lithium carbonate 0.4–2.0 g daily in divided doses depending on renal function and drug–plasma levels achieved.

Other drugs used in mania

Phenothiazines and other antipsychotic major tranquillisers have long been used in the management of acute mania. Symptoms are controlled, but it is not clear whether the duration of the manic episode is reduced. These drugs are useful in the treatment of acute attacks.

Chlorpromazine or haloperidol have been used successfully and may be used in combination with lithium carbonate.

Adverse effects are those of the dopamine receptor blocking and anticholinergic properties of these drugs particularly drug-induced Parkinsonian or dystonic reactions (Chapter 18.4).

Comment

Lithium carbonate is used for long-term prophylaxis in mania, and together with phenothiazines for control of symptoms in acute attacks. The daily dose of lithium depends on renal function and should be individually determined. Monitoring of lithium plasma levels is essential for optimal treatment without unacceptable adverse effects.

18.6 DRUG-INDUCED PSYCHIATRIC DISEASE

Central nervous system adverse effects of drugs are common especially in the case of lipid soluble drugs with specific effects either on:
(1) Receptors,

(2) Transmitter synthesis,
(3) Degradation of transmitters,
(4) Electrophysiological effects on excitable membranes.

A careful history of recent drug ingestion is an essential feature of the evaluation of a patient with psychiatric illness and where possible the first step in management of drug-induced psychiatric symptoms should be withdrawal of the offending drug.

There are many well documented examples of drugs causing behavioural adverse effects, which are summarised in Table 18.4.

TABLE 18.4   Drug-induced psychiatric disease

DEPRESSION

(1) *Antihypertensives*
Methyldopa
Clonidine
Reserpine
Propranolol
Guanethidine

(2) *Sedatives*
Barbiturates
Ethanol
Benzodiazepines

(3) *Neuroleptics*
Phenothiazines and
other antipsychotics

(4) *Steroids*
Corticosteroids
Oral contraceptive pill

(5) *Analgesics*
Opiates
Non-steroidal anti-
inflammatory drugs

(6) *Others*
Levodopa
Tetrabenazine
Methysergide

ORGANIC PSYCHOSIS

(1) Sympathomimetics (amphetamine)
(2) Beta-adrenoceptor antagonists (propranolol, oxprenolol)
(3) Anticholinergic drugs (atropine, benzhexol)
(4) Levodopa and dopamine agonists (bromocriptine, apomorphine)
(5) Steroids (prednisolone, dexamethasone)

ANXIETY AND ANXIETY SYMPTOMS

(1) Sympathomimetics (amphetamine, ephedrine, phenylpropanolamine, etc.)
(2) Beta$_2$-adrenoceptor agonists (isoprenaline, salbutamol, terbutaline)
(3) Drug withdrawal states (clonidine, barbiturates, opiates, alcohol)

18.7 ABUSE OF PSYCHOACTIVE DRUGS

Abuse of drugs and related agents has been noted with increased frequency in young people in urban communities. Less commonly, therapeutic drug use leads to dependence, e.g. opiate analgesic abuse in patients first treated for chronic severe pain. However, the concept of drug misuse or abuse must be judged in a cultural and historical context. Attitudes to non-therapeutic use of cannabis and even opiates differ greatly throughout the world.

The problems of drug abuse are:

(1) The direct specific toxic effects, e.g. respiratory depression with opiates.

(2) Generalised actions on mood, disinhibition of social behaviour, and impaired level of consciousness.

(3) Short-term consequences of drug withdrawal, e.g. psychological and physical symptoms of dependence.

(4) Long-term medical complications of the contemporary drug 'subculture', e.g. hepatitis, septicaemia, bacterial endocarditis.

Psychoactive drugs, like analgesics or sedatives, have a high potential for abuse because:

(1) *Central effects.* They modify mood or behaviour leading to either pleasurable experiences, depersonalisation or intoxication and unconsciousness.

(2) *Tolerance.* If there is tolerance to the effect with regular use and thus a need to increase the dose to get the same effect, then not only is the drug-taking habit reinforced but there is a greater risk of chemical toxicity or adverse effects at the higher doses.

(3) *Withdrawal symptoms.* Symptoms on withdrawal of the abused drug further reinforce the need for continued drug use (or abuse). While these withdrawal symptoms may often be psychological, in the case of opiates and barbiturates physical symptoms on withdrawal create further dependence or 'addiction'.

Drugs with a high abuse potential can be divided into:

(1) *Therapeutic agents*:
    (a) Benzodiazepines,
    (b) Barbiturates,
    (c) Other hypnotics and sedatives,
    (d) Antidepressants,
    (e) Opiate analgesics and analogues, including dextropropoxyphene.

(2) *Non-therapeutic agents* ('street' drugs)
  (a) Cannabis,
  (b) Cocaine,
  (c) Opiates,
  (d) Amphetamine, their therapeutic use now is very limited,
  (e) L S D, psyllocibin, phencyclidine and other hallucinogens,
  (f) Solvents,
  (g) Alcohol.

Comment

The management of drug abuse is not easy and involves:
  (1) Management of acute pharmacological toxicity.
  (2) Treatment of any acute medical complications, e.g. septicaemia, endocarditis.
  (3) Psychiatric assessment and treatment of any underlying psychopathology.
  (4) Controlled planned withdrawal of the drug, if necessary, with temporary substitution, e.g. methadone for heroin.
  (5) Long-term measures such as family or community support (Alcoholics Anonymous) psychotherapy or drug therapy (disulfiram for alcoholics).

CHAPTER 19

Drugs and neurological disease

19.1 Epilepsy

19.2 Extrapyramidal diseases

19.3 Migraine

19.4 Myasthenia gravis

19.1 EPILEPSY

Aim

Drug treatment should suppress generalised or focal seizures, without impairment of consciousness or motor function.

Relevant pathophysiology

Epilepsy is a paroxysmal disorder of brain function involving bursts of uncontrolled electrical activity. Epilepsy may be:
(1) Generalised
   (a) Primary
      (i) Grand mal, tonic-clonic seizures,
      (ii) petit mal, 'little absences' especially prevalent in children,
   (b) Secondary to tumour or infection.
(2) Partial
   (a) Simple, Jacksonian motor epilepsy
   (b) Complex, temporal lobe (psychomotor epilepsy)

Epileptic fits or convulsions must be distinguished from other causes of loss of consciousness, as treatment differs. A detailed history and description by the patient and witnesses is most useful, and may follow the classical 'march' of Jacksonian motor epilepsy, or the progression of a grand mal convulsion from aura, loss of consciousness, through tonic and clonic phases to post ictal drowsiness and weakness.

Epilepsy is a symptom not a pathological diagnosis. It is important to determine if epilepsy is primary, or secondary to head injury, tumour or other neurological disease.

Principles of drug treatment

Treatment must be as simple as possible and should be initiated with a single agent given in a dose which achieves therapeutic plasma levels. If one drug is not successful then a second drug may be substituted or added.

The choice of anticonvulsant depends on the type of epilepsy:

(1) Tonic-clonic seizures:
    (a) Phenytoin,
    (b) Sodium valproate,
    (c) Carbamazepine,
    (d) Phenobarbitone.

(2) Temporal lobe epilepsy:
    (a) Carbamazepine,
    (b) Phenytoin,
    (c) Phenobarbitone,
    (d) Sodium valproate.

(3) Jacksonian motor epilepsy:
    (a) Carbamazepine,
    (b) Phenytoin,
    (c) Sodium valproate,

(4) Petit mal:
    (a) Sodium valproate,
    (b) Ethosuximide.

Monitoring of plasma drug concentration is particularly useful in the management of epilepsy because:

(1) Therapeutic range of effective plasma levels has been defined for most anticonvulsants.

(2) Most anticonvulsants are metabolised by the liver and their

elimination varies in the population and is modified by enzyme inducers and inhibitors (Chapter 1).

(3) Compliance is often poor in epileptics.

Comment

Thereapeutic drug monitoring is essential if there are problems with fit control or suspected toxic reactions, and most useful with phenytoin and phenobarbitone, where the therapeutic range has been best defined.

Phenytoin

Mechanism

Phenytoin has direct effects to prevent the propagation of abnormal activity in neuronal membranes and other excitable tissues. It also has effects on turnover of gamma amino butyric acid (GABA), an inhibitory neurotransmitter. Phenytoin does not usually cause sedation if the plasma concentration is maintained within the optimal therapeutic range.

Pharmacokinetics

Phenytoin is well absorbed and its metabolism by the liver is capacity limited and binding sensitive (Chapter 2). Phenytoin differs from most other drugs in that the enzyme that metabolises it can be saturated when the dose is in the therapeutic range. This leads to a non-linear relationship between dose and plasma concentration within the therapeutic range. Non-linear or zero-order kinetics (see Chapter 5) cause unpredictable changes in plasma levels, the need for fine dose titration and above all careful monitoring of plasma concentration. The therapeutic range is 40–80 μmol/l (10–20 μg/ml). Phenytoin is extensively protein bound and in the presence of reduced protein binding the therapeutic range may have to be revised to a lower level (Chapter 2).

Adverse effects

These are numerous and may occur at:
(1) Therapeutic drug levels:
　(a) Gum hypertrophy,

(b) Hirsutism and acne,
(c) Lymphadenopathy,
(d) Skin rashes,
(e) Drug-induced lupus syndrome,
(f) Vitamin D deficiency ⎫ related to effects on
(g) Folic acid deficiency and ⎬ vitamin D and folate
(h) Megaloblastic anaemia ⎭ metabolism in the liver.
(2) At high plasma levels:
   (a) Nystagmus,
   (b) Ataxia,
   (c) Diplopia,
   (d) Nausea and vomiting,
   (e) Sedation,
   (f) Personality change,
   (g) Increased seizure frequency.

Drug interactions

Phenytoin metabolism may be impaired by drugs that inhibit liver enzymes. The following agents cause phenytoin to accumulate and may precipitate toxicity:
(1) Isoniazid,
(2) Sulthiame,
(3) Chloramphenicol,
(4) Sulphonamides.

Phenytoin metabolism can be induced with resulting low plasma levels and loss of therapeutic effect by:
(1) Carbamazepine,
(2) Alcohol,
(3) Steroids

Phenytoin can induce its own metabolism and that of other drugs, e.g. the contraceptive pill, with loss of efficacy (see Chapter 14).

Dose

Phenytoin: 150–400 mg (average 300 mg) once daily with individual titration using clinical response and plasma drug levels.

Comment

Phenytoin is a useful drug for treatment of grand mal seizures and focal epilepsy. Frequent adverse effects at toxic drug levels demand careful individual titration of drug dose, measurement of drug levels and maintenance of these within the narrow therapeutic range.

Sodium valproate

Mechanism

It elevates brain levels of the inhibitory transmitter gamma amino butyric acid (GABA) by preventing breakdown and uptake into nerve terminals. Valproate is increasingly used in the treatment not only of petit mal, but also of grand mal and focal epilepsy. It is relatively free of sedative effects.

Pharmacokinetics

Sodium valproate is well absorbed, metabolised by the liver and extensively protein bound (> 90%). Half-life is short (8–12 h). Therapeutic range 350–700 μmol/l (50–100 μg/ml) is not so well defined as for phenytoin.

Adverse effects

    (1) Nausea and gastric irritation,
    (2) Transient hair loss,
    (3) Thrombocytopenia,
    (4) Oedema,
    (5) Drug-induced hepatitis.

Dose

Sodium valproate: 200 mg two or three times daily increasing if necessary to maximum daily dose of 2.4–3.0 g.

Comment

Sodium valproate is a relatively new anticonvulsant. It is increasingly used in all types of epilepsy alone or in combination, as central adverse effects are not commonly troublesome.

Phenobarbitone

Mechanism

Widely used for over 60 years, long-acting barbiturates like phenobarbitone, have widespread non-specific depressant effects on neuronal membranes. These effects which have been exploited therapeutically (Chapter 18) must now be viewed as the major drawback to the use of these drugs in grand mal and focal epilepsy. Sedation and drowsiness overlap with their anticonvulsant properties at therapeutic levels. Primidone is metabolised to phenobarbitone. Its anticonvulsant action depends on the formation of phenobarbitone, and it has no advantages over the active agent.

Pharmacokinetics

Phenobarbitone is metabolised by hepatic enzymes and in part eliminated unchanged by the kidney. Phenobarbitone induces hepatic drug metabolising enzyme activity. The plasma half-life is long (50–90 h) permitting once daily dosing, usually at night.

Steady state levels may not be reached for 4–6 weeks. Therapeutic plasma levels lie between 80–100 μmol/l (15–20 μg/ml).

Adverse effects

(1) Sedation and drowsiness especially early in treatment,
(2) Vertigo, ataxia, headache,
(3) Behavioural changes, irritability and impaired learning (in children),
(4) Skin rashes,
(5) Elevation of plasma levels of liver transaminase enzyme activity,
(6) Dependence (psychological and possibly physical),
(7) Withdrawal reaction, including an increased frequency of fits.

Drug interactions

Hepatic enzyme induction may lead to changes in metabolism and effect of other metabolised drugs and vice versa. Caution is necessary when the dose of phenobarbitone is changed in patients on:

(1) Oral anticoagulants, warfarin,
(2) Oral contraceptive,
(3) Other anticonvulsants,
(4) Oral hypoglycaemic agents, tolbutamide.

Dose

90 mg (children) $\left.\right\}$ as a single evening dose
100–240 mg (adults)

Comment

Phenobarbitone is not now first choice treatment for generalised or focal epilepsy in view of the common short-term sedation and long-term behavioural effects.

Carbamazepine

Carbamazepine is an effective drug in grand mal epilepsy and is the drug of choice in focal temporal lobe epilepsy. It is also used in trigeminal neuralgia.

Pharmacokinetics

Extensively metabolised by the liver, it is a powerful enzyme inducer and can induce its own metabolism. It has a short plasma half-life (10 h). Plasma concentrations can be measured but the therapeutic range (3–12 μg/ml) is not so well established as that for phenytoin possibly because of the formation of active metabolites.

Adverse effects

(1) Nausea and vomiting,
(2) Diarrhoea,
(3) Dizziness and drowsiness especially when combined with benzodiazepines, phenytoin or barbiturates,
(4) Antidiuretic effect,
(5) Skin rash with photosensitivity,
(6) Drug-induced hepatitis,
(7) Agranulocytosis (rarely).

Dose

100–200 mg twice daily increasing to 1.2–1.6 g daily if required to maintain therapeutic plasma levels or to control fits.

Comment

Carbamazepine is a useful drug both in focal and grand mal epilepsy. It can be used alone or in combination with another anticonvulsants.

Other anticonvulsants

Ethosuximide is now the second choice, to sodium valproate, in treatment of petit mal. Adverse effects include mood change, drowsiness and gastrointestinal intolerance. Rarely, blood dyscrasias and drug-induced lupus. Given in divided doses of 500–1500 mg daily. Therapeutic range is between 40–80 μg/ml.

Benzodiazepines. These are useful in status epilepticus when given parenterally. In grand mal and petit mal although oral clonazepam is effective, sedative properties are marked and limit its use. Benzodiazepines, with or without steroids or ACTH, may be of value in infantile spasms (hypsarrhythmia).

Sulthiame is probably inactive as an anticonvulsant but may potentiate the effects of phenytoin, phenobarbitone or carbamazepine by inhibiting hepatic mixed function oxidases and increasing plasma levels of the active anticonvulsant drugs.

Treatment of status epilepticus

Status epilepticus is the continuous clinical manifestation of an epileptic discharge without intermission. Grand mal epilepsy with recurrent tonic–clonic convulsions without recovery of consciousness is a medical emergency requiring urgent treatment. Control of fits should be achieved as quickly as possible using either:

(1) **Diazepam** intravenously, 10 mg as a single dose followed by intravenous infusion of diazepam (100 mg in 500 ml of normal saline or glucose) titrated to control fits (about 1 mg/min).

(2) **Clonazepam**, another benzodiazepine, is an alternative as 1 mg intravenously or up to 3 mg by slow intravenous infusion.

(3) **Chlormethiazole** by intravenous infusion of the 0.8% solution (8 mg/ml) at a rate of 10–20 mg/min titrated to control fits.

(4) **Phenytoin** by intravenous injection can be used acutely to control fits if an appropriately high loading dose (1 g) is given. Subsequent doses are chosen after plasma level measurement.

(5) **Paraldehyde** given by deep intramuscular injection into the buttocks (10 ml each side) may still be useful in the emergency treatment of status epilepticus when there is difficulty with intravenous access. Paraldehyde is safe although the injection site may be painful and sterile abscesses may develop later. Glass syringes are advised as some but not all plastics are dissolved by paraldehyde.

Rarely if these manoeuvres do not control status epilepticus paralysis by curarisation and artificial ventilation may be required.

General measures include maintenance of an airway, administration of oxygen and regular observation of neurological and cardiorespiratory functions as for any unconscious patient, together with maintenance of fluid and electrolyte balance.

TABLE 19.1 Anticonvulsants: summary of indications, therapeutic ranges and doses

Drug	Indications	Therapeutic range	Dose range
Sodium valproate	Tonic clonic seizures, Petit mal	350–700 μmol/l 50–100 μg/ml	30–60 mg/kg/day 1800–4200 mg/day
Phenytoin	Tonic clonic seizures	40–80 μmol/l 10–20 μg/ml	5–6 mg/kg/day 300–400 mg/day
Carbamazepine	Tonic clonic seizures Temporal lobe	20–50 μmol/l 5–12 μg/ml	10–20 mg/kg/day 600–1400 mg/day
Phenobarbitone	Tonic clonic seizures	50–150 μmol/l 12–35 μg/ml	2–4 mg/kg/day 120–180 mg/day
Ethosuximide	Petit mal	284–710 μmol/l 40–100 μg/ml	20–30 mg/kg/day 1200–2100 mg/day

Comment

Drug treatment of epilepsy requires close co-operation between the patient, family doctor and neurologist or physician. The choice of drug depends on the type of epilepsy. Control of fits without impairment of consciousness, motor functions or behavioural disturbances is the goal of treatment. This is best achieved by:

(1) Simple regimens, one drug once a day if possible,

(2) Avoiding adverse effects or toxicity,

(3) Counselling to improve compliance,

(4) Monitoring plasma drug levels to maintain therapeutic concentrations.

19.2 EXTRAPYRAMIDAL DISEASES— PARKINSONISM

Aim

To replace brain dopamine deficiency in the striatum and restore motor function while minimising neurological, psychiatric and cardiovascular adverse effects of treatment.

Relevant pathophysiology

Parkinsonism is most common in older age groups (55 years +) and is characterised by:

(1) Tremor at rest (pill rolling type),

(2) Rigidity (lead pipe or cog wheel type),

(3) Hypokinesia (paucity of spontaneous movement).

These are associated with a loss of a dopamine containing neuronal pathway from the substantia nigra to the corpus striatum and low dopamine levels in the striatum.

A Parkinsonian syndrome may result from:

(1) Idiopathic nigrostriatal degeneration—common,

(2) Post-encephalitic—after viral infection,

(3) Drug induced

(a) phenothiazines and other antipsychotic drugs are dopamine receptor blockers,

(b) Other drugs: methyldopa, reserpine, tetrabenazine, deplete striatal dopamine,

(4) Other rarer causes include:

(a) Manganese poisoning,

(b) Carbon monoxide poisoning,

(c) Cerebrovascular disease,

(d) Wilson's Disease.

Principles of drug treatment

Parkinsonism results neurochemically from:
   (1) Absolute loss of dopamine in striatum,
   (2) Relative increase in the actions of acetylcholine in basal ganglia,
Rational drug treatment thus consists of restoring the dopaminergic–cholinergic balance in the striatum by:
   (1) Increasing dopamine effects, e.g. levodopa, bromocriptine,
   (2) Blocking acetylcholine actions, e.g. anticholinergics.
Although those with mild disease may start on anticholinergic drugs, the major disability of Parkinsonian patients is hypokinesia with difficulty walking, dressing and eating. When this appears, levodopa is given, often in addition to anticholinergics.
   Physiotherapy, occupational therapy and social support are important adjuncts to treatment but stereotactic surgery has very little place nowadays.

Levodopa

Mechanism

The immediate precursor of dopamine in catecholamine synthesis, levedopa is decarboxylated in the brain to replenish striatal dopamine. Dopamine itself cannot be given as it is not absorbed by mouth and does not cross the blood–brain barrier. Adverse effects of levodopa result from the effects of dopamine and other active amines formed in the brain and periphery. Levodopa is now used together with a peripheral, or extracerebral, decarboxylase inhibitor, carbidopa or benserazide. Peripheral decarboxylase inhibitors block levodopa formation from levodopa *outside* the brain, but are polar drugs, which themselves *do not cross* the blood–brain barrier and thus do not influence brain decarboxylation.
   Peripheral decarboxylation inhibitors:
   (1) Prevent extracerebral adverse effects due to formation of catecholamines:
      (a) Arrhythmias,
      (b) Hypertension,
      (c) Nausea and vomiting.
   (2) Reduce the daily dose of levodopa required.

Pharmacokinetics

Levodopa is absorbed from the jejunum and may compete with dietary aromatic amino acids. It has a short plasma half-life (1–2 h), but in many patients it can be given twice or three times daily. However, long-term treatment may lead to dramatic changes in performance which are improved by smaller, more frequent doses.

Adverse effects

These result from the pharmacological effects of dopamine, noradrenaline and metabolites. They are usually dose related. Psychiatric adverse effects may require drug withdrawal:

(1) Dyskinesia, new involuntary movements, commonly dose limiting,

(2) On–off fluctuations in performance particularly with long-term (> 5 year) treatment,

(3) Psychiatric effects, e.g. psychosis, depression or mania,

(4) Postural hypotension,

(5) Nausea and vomiting, early in treatment, worse on levodopa alone,

(6) Cardiac arrhythmias, especially with levodopa alone,

(7) Open angle glaucoma,

Clinical use and dose

Levodopa and carbidopa (Sinemet), and levodopa and benserazide (Madopar).

Tablets: two or three (or more) times daily in an individually *titrated dose*: starting at 200–300 mg of levodopa and increasing up to 1 g daily of levodopa.

Comment

Levodopa dose must be individually titrated to obtain the maximum improvement in motor function while minimising adverse effects. The efficacy of levodopa falls off with long-term treatment indicating that the underlying neurological disease progresses and is not reversed by levodopa treatment.

Anticholinergic drugs

Mechanism

Synthetic atropine-like drugs that competitively block the muscarinic cholinergic receptor. Several are available including:
(1) Benzhexol,
(2) Benztropine,
(3) Orphenadrine.
Modest therapeutic effect in Parkinsonism with improvement in rigidity. Dose increased to maximum tolerated without adverse effects. Usually used together with levodopa preparations or alone in mild early disease. There are few differences between anticholinergics and no justification for using more than one drug from this group at any time.

Adverse effects

Adverse effects are those of blockade of muscarinic cholinergic receptors.
(1) Central nervous system, e.g. confusion, disorientation, sedation and rarely psychosis
(2) Cardiovascular, e.g. tachycardia, arrhythmias.
(3) Gastrointestinal, e.g. dry mouth, constipation
(4) Urinary, e.g. hesitancy, frequency.
(5) Paralysis of visual accommodation and glaucoma.

Doses

Benzhexol	2–15 mg	Daily in two or more divided
Benztropine	100–400 mg	doses starting at low levels
Orphenadrine	0.5–4 mg	and increasing if tolerated

    Benztropine and orphenadrine can be given intravenously or intramuscularly in the treatment of drug-induced dystonia.

Other antiParkinsonian drugs

Amantadine has modest antiParkinsonian effects. It is relatively free of adverse effects but may cause confusion if given at night. It can be tried in patients who cannot tolerate levodopa. It has also antiviral activity (Chapter 9.5). The beneficial effect of long term amantadine is disputed.

Bromocriptine is a direct dopamine receptor agonist, which has a similar range of actions and at least as severe adverse effects as levodopa. It has no clear advantage over levodopa in the majority of patients. The clinical pharmacology of bromocriptine is described in Chapter 20.2.

Drug-induced extrapyramidal symptoms

Most commonly seen following phenothiazines in the treatment of schizophrenia and other psychosis. Also after anti-emetics with dopamine receptor blocking properties, e.g. prochlorperazine, metoclopramide.

The symptoms occurring depend on the age of the patient:
(1) Parkinsonian syndrome, in older patients,
(2) Acute dystonic reactions, in younger patients,
(3) Tardive dyskinesia (Chapter 18.4).

Levodopa should not be given for drug-induced Parkinsonism.

Treatment is by reduction in dose or cessation of the drug if possible. Alternatively long-term anticholinergic drugs (benztropine or benzhexol) may be given. Acute dystonic reactions respond rapidly to intravenous benztropine or orphenadrine.

Chorea

Chorea, either Huntingdon's, the familial form, or secondary to cerebrovascular damage in the basal ganglia is characterised by repetitive semi-purposive movements which resemble levedopa-induced dyskinesia.

The neurochemistry of chorea is not established, but functionally may include overactivity of dopamine systems in the basal ganglia due to deficiency of the inhibitory transmitter GABA.

Chorea may be treated with:
(1) **Tetrabenazine**, which depletes dopamine from nerve endings. Adverse side effects are sedation, depression and Parkinsonism.
(2) **Haloperidol** (a butyrophenone) or **phenothiazines**, which act as dopamine receptor blockers and cause Parkinsonism or dystonic reactions as common adverse effects.
(3) **Sodium valproate**, which elevates brain levels of GABA.

Comment

Treatment of extrapyramidal diseases involves the adjustment of the level of cholinergic and dopaminergic activity in the basal ganglia. This requires increasing dopamine effects in Parkinsonism and reducing dopamine effects in chorea.

Adverse effects result both from over correction of the local transmitter function and more distant consequences on other brain and peripheral receptors of modification of neurotransmitter function.

19.3 MIGRAINE

Headache is a frequent symptom which, rarely, is caused by underlying neurological disease and is most often ascribed to 'tension'. Treatment is usually symptomatic often by self medication with 'over the counter' preparations.

Relevant pathophysiology

Migraine is a specific, common, often familial, form of vascular headache. Onset in older patients (>40 years) may suggest an underlying cerebral lesion (tumour or vascular malformation). If symptoms begin at a younger age no underlying cause is usually found.

Characteristically an attack of migraine consists of:

(1) A premonitory period of listlessness, often with visual disturbance and flashing lights or focal neurological features lasting up to 30 min.

(2) A unilateral headache spreading from behind the eye. The headache is constant and throbbing, and may be accompanied by photophobia, nausea and vomiting. It may last 6–12 h or rarely for several days.

The initial aura and warning symptoms or focal neurological features are believed to be caused by vasoconstriction of intracranial blood vessels while the later headache is the result of vasodilatation of extracerebral and intracerebral vessels. Migraine may be provoked by humoral agents, vasoactive amines, prostaglandins or peptides in a proportion of patients. Tyramine or tyramine-containing foods may precipitate headaches in some patients with migraine. The therapeutic efficacy of serotonin antagonists suggests that serotonin may also contribute.

Principles of drug treatment

Management of migraine consists of:
(1) Avoidance of precipitating factors, e.g. cheese, chocolate, meat extract, or alcohol.
(2) Symptomatic treatment of the acute attack with simple analgesics. Ergotamine preparations, bed rest and anti-emetics are required in more severe cases.
(3) Prophylactic treatment if the frequency of attacks justifies it with serotonin antagonists (pizotifen) or beta-receptor blockers (propranolol).

Ergotamine

Still widely used for the management of the more severe attacks. Ergot alkaloids are alpha-receptor blockers and also have direct vascular effects causing vasoconstriction. Thus they can modify the constriction and dilatation believed to underlie the symptoms. Ergotamine may also block serotonin receptors.
Ergotamine is given during the prodromal phase of the migraine attack either:
(1) Sublingually,
(2) Rectally by suppository,
(3) Subcutaneously or intramuscularly,
(4) By aerosol nebuliser.
Gastrointestinal irritation together with migraine induced nausea and vomiting and gastric stasis make oral dosing of little use.
Ergotamine may be given together with an anti-emetic.

Adverse effects

(1) Nausea and vomiting,
(2) Abdominal pain and cramps,
(3) Withdrawal headache,
(4) Peripheral vasoconstriction with Raynaud's phenomenon in patients with coexisting peripheral vascular disease.
Ergotamine is contraindicated in pregnancy and in patients with cerebrovascular or peripheral vascular disease.

Clinical use and dose

Ergotamine tartrate: *Sublingually*: 1–2 mg to a total dose of 6–8 mg per attack or 12 mg/week.
Rectally: 2 mg repeated after 1 h to same total dose as above.
By aerosol: 360 μg inhalation repeated up to six inhalations daily or 15 per week.

Metoclopramide may be used in the management of an acute attack of migraine both to prevent nausea and vomiting (Chapter 15.3) and to speed gastric emptying and facilitate absorption of orally administered analgesics.

Comment

Ergotamine is used for treatment of the acute attack and *never* prophylactically. Proprietary preparations often contain caffeine, analgesics, or anti-emetics.

Other drugs used in treatment of migraine

Pizotifen is now the prophylactic treatment of choice. This serotonin receptor antagonist also has anticholinergic properties.
Adverse effects include drowsiness, weight gain and dizziness. It is given orally as 0.5 mg twice or three times daily in long term to reduce the frequency of acute migraine attacks.

Propranolol A non-selective beta-receptor blocker has been found to reduce the frequency of migraine attacks in many patients. It is given orally in daily doses of 40–80 mg. Adverse effects are discussed in Chapter 9.

Diazepam or other benzodiazepines may be useful if anxiety appears to be a precipitating factor.

Clonidine The alpha$_2$-receptor agonist, used in much lower dose (50–100 μg) than to treat hypertension, has been claimed to reduce the frequency of attacks.

Methysergide is a serotonin receptor blocker, which although effective may lead to retroperitoneal fibrosis with long-term use and should only be considered in severe cases resistant to other agents.

Comment

Migraine prophylaxis depends on avoidance of identified precipitating factors and if required long-term treatment with pizotifen or propranolol as prophylaxis to reduce the frequency of acute attacks.

Acute attacks are controlled by simple analgesics supplemented if required by ergotamine and anti-emetics.

19.4 MYASTHENIA GRAVIS

Relevant pathophysiology

Myasthenia gravis is a disease of the muscle motor end plate resulting in impaired cholinergic transmission. There is now evidence of an immunological basis with circulating antibodies to the cholinergic receptor and a reduction in the numbers of cholinergic receptors contributing to fluctuating motor weakness.

Muscles of the orbit are commonly affected leading to ptosis and diplopia. Other facial and limb girdle muscles may be involved. Respiratory muscle involvement may rarely require artificial ventilation. Diagnosis is based on history of fatigue of motor responses, recovery with rest and a therapeutic response to an anticholinesterase drug.

Principles of drug treatment

Treatment of myasthenia aims at increasing the availability of acetylcholine at the motor end plate. This is achieved by preventing the breakdown of acetylcholine by blockade of acetylcholinesterase with neostigmine or pyridostigmine. The dose of anticholinesterase drug is titrated to give optimal performance. Weakness can result not only from lack of acetylcholine (myasthenic weakness) but also from excess acetylcholine (cholinergic weakness) due to a depolarisation block of the motor end plate. These can be distinguished using a test dose of edrophonium, a short acting anticholinesterase.

Neostigmine and pyridostigmine

Mechanism

These have structural similarities to the substrate, acetylcholine and act as competitive (reversible) antagonists of cholinesterase enzymes. They are slowly hydrolysed with recovery of cholinesterase activity. Pyridostigmine has the longer duration of action. They are given orally or by subcutaneous, intramuscular or intravenous injection. The oral dose is titrated individually to optimise motor response without cholinergic crises of persistent depolarisation.

Adverse effects

These are symptoms and signs of muscarinic cholinergic overactivity:
(1) Nausea and vomiting,
(2) Increased salivation,
(3) Sweating,
(4) Spontaneous defaecation and micturition,
(5) Miosis,
(6) Bradycardia and hypotension,
(7) Agitation,
(8) Muscle fasciculation.

Many of these symptoms can be controlled by atropine-like drugs, which block the muscarinic cholinergic receptor. Atropine or propantheline may be given together with neostigmine.

Drug interactions

Weakness may be precipitated by aminoglycoside antibiotics including streptomycin and gentamicin, which have neuromuscular blocking properties and also phenytoin and phenothiazines. Myasthenic patients are especially sensitive to neuromuscular blocking agents.

Clinical use and dose

Neostigmine: *Orally*: 75–300 mg daily in titrated divided doses.
Parenterally: 2–5 mg daily in divided doses.
Pyridostigmine: *Orally*: 0.3–1.2 g daily in titrated divided doses.
Parenterally: 2–5 mg daily in divided doses.

Other approaches to the treatment of myasthenia

Steroids or immunosuppressant therapy have been used to induce a remission in the fluctuating course of myasthenia that is not responding adequately to anticholinesterase treatment. Patients may deteriorate early in a course of steroids and may require temporary artificial ventilation. ACTH may be used as an alternative to steroids.

Plasmapheresis has been reported in the short term to improve motor function, presumably by removing humoral antibodies or other circulating immune mediators. Plasmapheresis is currently used in the preparation of patients with severe disease for thymectomy.

Thymectomy may induce remission, particularly in younger women. Up to 80% of patients may be in remission 3–5 years after surgery.

Comment

Treatment of myasthenia aims to maximise motor power and performance without inducing depolarisation block or muscarinic adverse effects of overdose.

CHAPTER 20

Drugs and endocrine disease

20.1   DIABETES MELLITUS

Aims

The purpose is to restore metabolism to normal and prevent both short-term complications, e.g. infection and ketoacidosis, and long-term consequences, e.g. retinopathy, neuropathy, etc., of diabetes mellitus.

Relevant pathophysiology

Diabetes mellitus is characterised by:

(1) Deranged secretion of insulin and glucagon with extensive disturbance of carbohydrate, protein and lipid metabolism.

(2) Thickening of capillary basement membranes throughout the body.

(3) Long-term complications involving the eye, kidney, peripheral nervous system and circulation.

Therapy is aimed directly or indirectly at the deranged secretion of insulin and thereby at correcting the metabolic abnormalities. Diabetes mellitus encompasses a wide variation both in the secretion of insulin and in concentration of insulin receptors at the target cell membrane. At one extreme, non-insulin dependent (usually obese) diabetics have high serum insulin concentrations and low insulin receptor concentrations. These high absolute insulin concentrations still represent a deficiency in relative terms when serum glucose is taken into account. If an obese hyperinsulinaemic individual loses weight then both serum insulin and receptor concentration return toward normal with a consequent improvement in glucose homeostasis. The opposite extreme is represented by the insulin-dependent diabetic who has extremely low or immeasurable serum insulin concentrations because of irreversible loss of functioning pancreatic beta cells. In the first type of patient, treatment is aimed at optimising the secretion and effect of the body's own insulin. For the second type of patient, replacement therapy with insulin is necessary.

Insulin

Mechanism

The major actions of insulin are inhibition of gluconeogenesis and increasing uptake of glucose by muscle and fat cells.

In addition, insulin potentiates:
(1) Conversion of glucose to glycogen,
(2) Conversion of aminoacids to proteins,
(3) Conversion of glucose to fatty acids,
(4) Conversion of fatty acids to triglycerides.
Conversely, insulin inhibits these catabolic processes:
(1) Conversion of protein to aminoacids,
(2) Conversion of triglycerides to fatty acids.

Pharmacokinetics

Absorption Insulin is destroyed by gastrointestinal enzymes and therefore always given parenterally.

Elimination. Insulin is degraded in liver and kidney. Its half-life is about 9 minutes.

Adverse effects

The most frequent, and potentially most serious, is hypoglycaemia. This is usually precipitated by missing a meal, unaccustomed exercise or administering too much insulin. Early symptoms are visual disturbance, drowsiness, sweating, incoordination followed by hunger, weakness, anxiety, and tachycardia. More severe hypoglycaemia is associated with a wide range of neurological disturbance, including seizures and coma, and is a medical emergency. Minor and transient allergies can occur at the site of injection. Since the introduction of highly purified insulins atrophy of fat at injection sites and formation of antibodies to heterologous insulin have become very uncommon.

Drug interactions

The hypoglycaemic action of insulin can be prolonged by acute alcohol intoxication and by monoamine oxidase inhibition.

Beta-blockers can interact in three ways:

(1) Some warning signs of hypoglycaemia are masked by beta blockade, e.g. tachycardia and anxiety. However, sweating may be increased.

(2) Hypoglycaemia can be prolonged because adrenaline-induced glycogenolysis is impaired.

(3) The increased catecholamine release during hypoglycaemia can cause a marked rise in blood pressure by unopposed action on vascular alpha-receptors (the beta-receptors that mediate vasodilatation being blocked by drug).

All these interactions probably involve beta$_2$ receptors. If a diabetic on treatment is to receive a beta blocker this should be preferably beta$_1$ selective.

The effectiveness of insulin can be reduced by drugs with hyperglycaemic actions, e.g. thiazide diuretics, frusemide and corticosteroids.

Insulin formulations

The insulins currently used are obtained from beef or pork pancreas, but it is likely that recombinant DNA techniques will soon allow commercial production of insulin from bacteria. Improved preparation techniques have resulted in highly purified insulins becoming available in recent years. However, apart from avoidance of fat atrophy these new insulin preparations are of no proven advantage over conventional types.

TABLE 20.1 Insulin formulations

Duration of Action	Examples	Peak effect (h)	Duration of action (h)
Short	Insulin injection (Soluble insulin)	2–4	6–12
Intermediate	Isophane insulin	5–12	12–24
	Insulin zinc suspension (amorphous)	3–6	12–16
Long	Protamine zinc	5–14	24–30
Mixed	Biphasic (short + intermediate)	2–10	18–20
	Insulin zinc suspension (intermediate + long)	3–8	16–24

In order to prolong its biological action, insulin is given by subcutaneous injection thereby slowing its rate of delivery to the circulation. Absorption can be slowed further by combining the insulin with protamine (a basic protein) or zinc or both, the resulting preparation having a slower onset but longer duration of action. A further modification in rate of absorption depends on whether the insulin preparation is amorphous or crystalline, the latter dissolving more slowly. Broadly speaking, insulin preparations can be divided into four categories, (1) short, (2) intermediate, (3) long, and (4) mixed depending on their onset and duration of action following subcutaneous administration (Table 20.1).

Dose

Short-acting insulins are available in strengths of 20, 40, 80, 100 and 320 units/ml. Intermediate and long-acting insulins are available at 40 and 80 units/ml. The dose, frequency or administration and combination of insulin formulations used depend on numerous factors which vary greatly between individuals. A typical regimen would be soluble and isophane twice a day. The effectiveness of treatment has traditionally been assessed by home monitoring for glycosuria, but patient monitoring of blood glucose is being increasingly employed using capillary blood on glucose oxidase impregnated sticks. Adequacy of control can also be judged from the percentage of glycosylated haemoglobin.

Comment

Subcutaneous insulin cannot reproduce physiological levels and some success is being obtained with portable infusion pumps.

Oral hypoglycaemic drugs

Sulphonylureas

Mechanism

Sulphonylureas act primarily by stimulating pancreatic beta cells to produce more insulin. Functioning pancreatic tissue is, therefore, necessary for their action. In addition they inhibit both gluconeogenesis and insulin degradation in the liver and possibly increase insulin receptor density. An unrelated action of chlorpropamide and, to a lesser extent, tolbutamide is to increase the release and effect of antidiuretic hormone.

Pharmacokinetics

All sulphonylureas are effective following oral administration. The pharmacokinetic indices of sulphonylureas are summarised in Table 20.2. All except chlorpropamide are cleared by liver metabolism. There is a considerable range of half-life, some drugs being suitable for once daily dosing, e.g. chlorpropamide, while others, such as tolbutamide, must be given more frequently. Tolbutamide is extensively protein bound.

Adverse effects

All sulphonylureas can cause symptomatic hypoglycaemia which is the most frequent adverse reaction. Chlorpropamide can cause prolonged hypoglycaemia particularly when renal function is reduced, e.g. in old age. Much less frequently the sulphonylureas are associated with allergic reactions, mainly rashes, gastrointestinal symptoms, bone marrow suppression and cholestatic jaundice, which can be either allergic or dose related.

Glymidine is a sulphapyramidine and does not cross react with

TABLE 20.2 Sulphonylureas currently in clinical use

	Half-life (h)	Clearance route	Dose (mg)	Frequency of daily dose
Acetohexamide	2–5	M (A)	250	2–3
Chlorpropamide*	36	K	100–500	1
Glibenclamide	6	M	5	1–3
Glibornuride	8	M	12.5–75	1
Gliclazide	12	M	40–320	1
Glipizide	2–4	M	2.5–7.5	2–3
Gliquidone	1½	M	15–45	2–3
Glymidine	5–8	M (A)	500	1–3
Tolazamide	8	M (A)	100–500	1–2
Tolbutamide	5–8	M	500	2–4

M, metabolised by liver; K, excreted unchanged by kidney; A, active metabolites.
* A small proportion of chlorpropamide is metabolised to active products but renal elimination is the major route of clearance.

sulphonylureas if skin sensitivity occurs. There are two problems peculiar to chlorpropamide. First, though rarely, its antidiuretic effect can lead to worsening of heart failure. Second, a proportion of patients (up to one-third) experience flushing when they take alcohol. This is an autosomal dominant trait and may involve endogenous opioids since it is reversed by naloxone.

Drug interactions

The interactions described for insulin apply also to the sulphonylureas. Additional interactions include the following.

Tolbutamide: phenylbutazone and warfarin increase the hypoglycaemic effect both by inhibiting hepatic oxidation and by displacement from protein binding sites.

Chlorpropamide: high dose aspirin decreases renal excretion and therefore potentiates effect.

Clinical use and dose

One of the shorter acting sulphonylureas, such as tolbutamide, provides scope for flexibility in dosage to meet individual requirements (Table 20.2). However, a long-acting drug, e.g.

chlorpropamide, might be of benefit in improving compliance with therapy. Chlorpropamide should be avoided in elderly patients and those with renal or cardiac failure.

Biguanides (metformin and phenformin)

Mechanisms

Uncertain, but the following effects are likely to contribute:
(1) Decrease glucose absorption from the gut,
(2) Increase glucose entry to cells,
(3) Anorectic effect.

Pharmacokinetics

Metformin is excreted unchanged by the kidney. Phenformin is eliminated partly by hydroxylation and partly by the kidney. The hydroxylation of phenformin is genetically determined and approximately 10% of the population are poor metabolisers and may experience enhanced drug effect.

Adverse effects

Lactic acidosis is the most serious, though uncommon, problem. It carries a high mortality, is more common with phenformin and in patients with renal, hepatic or cardiac dysfunction. The more frequent adverse effects affect the gastrointestinal tract: nausea, vomiting and diarrhoea.

Drug interactions

The only interaction specific to biguanides is that tetracyclines can precipitate lactic acidosis in patients on phenformin.

Dose

Metformin: 0.5–1 g 8 hourly
Phenformin: 25 mg twice daily; this drug is now rarely used because of the risk of lactic acidosis.

Clinical use, benefits and risks of insulin and oral hypoglycaemic drugs

Most patients whose disease starts below the age of 40 years are insulin dependent, but a small proportion of those who develop diabetes later in life also require insulin. Sulphonylureas are second-line treatment for non-insulin dependent diabetics; diet is more important and drugs are used only when this has failed. Use of biguanides is declining though their anorectic effect is sometimes used in the refractory obese patient.

Treatment has well established benefits: prevention of ketoacidosis and death; alleviating symptoms such as polyuria and polydipsia; preventing infections. However, there is currently no clear evidence that treatment influences the long-term microvascular changes which result in blindness, renal failure and vascular disease.

The potential hazards of treatment described above are all avoidable. However, one large study (University Group Diabetes Program) suggested that tolbutamide-treated patients had a higher cardiovascular mortality than those on placebo. Evidence has subsequently been presented both to refute and support this finding, but this controversy strengthens the view that *weight loss* rather than drug treatment is the first choice management of obese non-insulin dependent diabetics.

Comment

The management of diabetes mellitus illustrates how a clear understanding of pathophysiology can have considerable impact on treatment. With high insulin concentration and low receptor number secondary to obesity it is quite illogical to give more insulin when a programme of weight reduction attacks the basic cause.

Treatment of diabetic emergencies

Hypoglycaemic coma

Causes. Coma is usually precipitated by missing a meal, unaccustomed exercise or taking too much insulin or sulphonylurea.

Clinical features. It can present with a wide range of neurological signs. *Every* medical emergency arriving with mental impairment, coma or other neurological signs *must* have a capillary glucose checked *on arrival*.

Treatment. 50 ml of 50% dextrose intravenously and repeat as necessary. Alternatively, glucagon 1 mg by intravenous or intramuscular route; useful if patient is difficult to restrain.

Ketoacidosis

This is an outline of a complex management problem.

Causes. Infections are the most common identifiable cause. Myocardial infarction, trauma and inadequate insulin dosage are other causes.

Clinical features. Typically these patients are dehydrated, hyperventilating and may have impaired consciousness. Serum glucose is usually markedly elevated and arterial pH is low.

Treatment. This is based on four measures:
(1) Fluid to replace dehydration,
(2) Insulin to control hyperglycaemia,
(3) Potassium to counter hypokalaemia,
(4) Bicarbonate to reverse metabolic acidosis.
Typical deficiencies would be: water 6 l; sodium 600 mmol (mEq); potassium 400 mmol (mEq).

Fluid: 1000 ml isotonic saline in 30 min.
      1000 ml isotonic saline in 1 h.
      1000 ml isotonic saline in 2 h.
      1000 ml isotonic saline in 4 h.
      500 ml isotonic saline 4 hourly.
Note: Use a central venous pressure line in the elderly or those with cardiac disease. If serum sodium rises above 155 mmol/l (mEq/l) use half normal saline.

Insulin. Soluble insulin 6 units/h by infusion pump. Double rate if glucose not falling at 2 h.
When blood glucose < 15 mmol/l (270 mg/100 ml) change to 5%

TABLE 20.3 Potassium regime.

mmol (mEq)/h	plasma K$^+$ mmol (mEq)/l
39	< 3
26	3–4
20	4–5
13	5–6
0	> 6

glucose infusion at the rate of 500 ml 4 hourly (add 13 mmol/l potassium chloride) and give insulin 3 units/h. Continue until patient is eating.

Potassium. Giving insulin and correcting acidosis lowers plasma potassium. Hypokalaemia is a *major* cause of morbidity in treating ketoacidosis. Give 20 mmol/h from the beginning, adjusting as shown in Table 20.3 for plasma potassium.

Continuous monitoring of the electrocardiogram should be undertaken; changes in T waves give early indication of important changes in plasma potassium.

Bicarbonate. If arterial blood pH < 7 give 100 mmol (mEq), sodium bicarbonate with 20 mmol (mEq), potassium chloride over 60 min. Repeat as indicated by monitoring pH.

Comment

Successful treatment of ketoacidosis depends on frequent monitoring of, and rapid response to, biochemical and haemodynamic data.

Remember that there is often an underlying cause. If you suspect infection, treat with antibiotics after relevant culture specimens have been obtained.

Hyperosmolar, non-ketotic hyperglycaemic coma

Cause is obscure. Usually found in the elderly or non-insulin dependent diabetics.

Features. Typical laboratory findings are very high blood glucose, raised urea, raised sodium and a high plasma osmolality.

Treatment

Isotonic saline, or half normal if plasma sodium > 150 mmol (mEq)/l. Adjust rate of infusion from a central venous pressure line. Give insulin as for ketoacidosis and possibly heparin as these patients are prone to thrombosis.

20.2 THYROID DISEASE

Hyperthyroidism

Aim

The purpose is to restore thyroid function to normal.

General

Drugs are used in the management of hyperthyroidism in three main ways:

(1) Interference with biosynthesis of thyroid hormones, e.g. carbimazole, methimazole or propylthiouracil. This aims to control thyroid overactivity while natural resolution occurs.

(2) Destruction of thyroid tissue, by radioactive iodine, which aims at limiting excess hormone production by ablating tissue.

(3) Interference with the peripheral effects of excess circulating hormone using beta-adrenoceptor blockade. This has as its goal purely symptomatic relief while other forms of treatment are being introduced.

Less common types of drug use are:

(4) Decreasing thyroid hormone release using potassium iodide.

(5) Interference with iodine trapping by the thyroid using potassium perchlorate.

Carbimazole, methimazole and propylthiouracil

Mechanism

These drugs act at three steps of thyroid hormone synthesis:

(1) Oxidation of iodide to iodine,

(2) Iodination of tyrosine,
(3) Coupling of iodotyrosines.
Secretion is not affected so their action is not apparent until hormone stores run down over 2–4 weeks.

Pharmacokinetics

Carbimazole is hydrolysed in plasma to methimazole and this is the active drug. Both methimazole and propylthiouracil are rapidly metabolised. Both drugs cross the placenta and enter breast milk to a clinically significant extent.

Adverse effects

The most common problem is hypothyroidism because of over-treatment. Another important, though rare, problem is agranulocytosis. Patients should be warned to report any sore throat or fever immediately. Rashes are common with carbimazole; arthralgia is rare.

Drug interactions

Propylthiouracil can cause hypoprothrombinaemia, which can interfere with anticoagulant dose.

Clinical use and dose

Carbimazole: 10 mg 8 hourly is the initial dose. Response is seen in 2–4 weeks, during which time thyroid gland hormone reserves are being depleted, and the dose is then slowly reduced to around 5 mg/day.
   Methimazole: 5–10 mg 8 hourly, reducing to 5–10 mg daily once control has been achieved. Current practice is to continue treatment for about a year. Permanent remission occurs in 50% of patients following the first course of treatment and a further 25% following a second course.
   Propylthiouracil: Initial dose is 100 mg 8 hourly with maintenance of 50–100 mg/day. Most often used in patients who develop a rash with carbimazole. In addition to the mechanisms listed above, propylthiouracil decreases peripheral conversion of T_4 to T_3 and this might contribute to its action.

Radioactive iodine (^{131}I)

The principle of this treatment is partial ablation of thyroid tissue by ^{131}I. Advantages are its simplicity (one dose taken orally) low cost and relative safety. Disadvantages are the difficulty in calculating correct dose and potential risk of genetic damage in women of childbearing age, who constitute the majority of hyperthyroid patients. ^{131}I is therefore given only to people beyond their reproductive years. The only major problem is hypothyroidism which develops at the rate of 10–15% in the first year and 3–6% per year thereafter.

Beta-adrenoceptor blockade

Several major symptoms of hyperthyroidism suggest increased sensitivity of peripheral beta-adrenoceptors to circulating catecholamines, though the exact mechanism remains uncertain. Administration of a beta-blocker can produce substantial symptomatic relief with reduction in tachycardia and tremor and a general decrease in anxiety. It must be emphasised that symptomatic relief is all that is achieved by beta-blockade; the underlying process is uninfluenced except for a modest reduction in peripheral conversion of T_4 to T_3. However, while waiting for carbimazole to take effect, or in preparation for surgery, beta-blocker therapy can be very useful. Propranolol is most commonly used, the dose being 40–80 mg twice daily.

Potassium iodide

This prevents hormone release from the gland. Main use is in thyroid crisis but occasionally used for 1–2 weeks in preparing patient for surgery.

Potassium perchlorate

This prevents uptake and concentrations of iodine by thyroid. Wide range of adverse reactions including aplastic anaemia. Used only if other treatment contraindicated.

Thyroid crisis

Clinical features are delirium, fever, tachycardia, dehydration and diarrhoea. It is a medical emergency. Treat with: rehydration, intravenous beta-blocker, potassium iodide, carbimazole and dexamethasone.

Hypothyroidism

General

Treatment is directed at replacement of the thyroid hormone deficiency. Two preparations are available: thyroxine (T_4) and triiodothyronine (T_3), although the latter is rarely used.

Mechanism

These preparations provide replacement therapy by stimulation of metabolism, growth and maturation.

Pharmacokinetics

Both T_4 and T_3 are adequately absorbed following oral administration. T_4 has a half-life of about a week and T_3 of about 2 days. Both undergo liver conjugation and enterohepatic circulation.

Adverse effects. These are related to physiological and pharmacological actions of thyroid hormone.

Elderly patients or those known to have ischaemic heart disease must receive low initial doses with slow increments since angina, infarction, tachyarrhythmias or heart failure can be precipitated. Excess dosage produces the features of hyperthyroidism.

Dose

Thyroxine: Starting dose is 0.05 mg/day (0.025 mg/day if old or with heart disease) with dose increments every 2–3 weeks depending on thyroid function.

20.3   CALCIUM METABOLISM

Vitamin D (calciferol)

Mechanism

Vitamin D is inactive. Its biological effect depends on hydroxylation at the 25 position in liver and 1 position in kidney to form 1,25 dihydroxycholecalciferol (1,25 DHCC). The major effect of 1,25 DHCC is mobilisation of calcium from bone and a less important action is to increase calcium reabsorption from kidney, leading to an increase of serum calcium.

Pharmacokinetics

Vitamin D is fat soluble and bile is necessary for absorption.

Adverse reactions

Hypercalcaemia and its consequences are the major problem; serum calcium should be monitored regularly during treatment.

Drug interactions

Anticonvulsants and other drugs can induce the enzymes which metabolise vitamin D and can produce deficiency states of rickets or osteomalacia.

Clinical use and dose

Calcium with vitamin D: Tablets BP contain, in addition to calcium salts, 12.5 μg of ergocalciferol and are used for prophylaxis and treatment of rickets and osteomalacia in the dose of 12.5–125 μg/day.

Calciferol tablets: High-strength BP contain cholecalciferol or ergocalciferol 250 μg and are used to treat resistant rickets or hypoparathyroidism in the dose of 1.25–3.75 mg/day.

1-α-Hydroxycholecalciferol

Mechanism

Hydroxylated to 1,25 DHCC in the liver.

Adverse effects

May cause hypercalcaemia and regular monitoring of serum calcium is essential.

Clinical use and dose

Renal rickets: 1 hydroxylation of vitamin D can be impaired in chronic renal failure. 1-α-HCC is given in the dose of 1 μg/day in addition to phosphate-binding drugs. PO_4 retention predisposes to hypocalcaemia with subsequent inappropriate elevation of parathyroid hormone levels.

Hypoparathyroidism: 1-α-HCC produces a more rapid response than vitamin D. Dose is 3–5 μg/day with calcium supplements.

Vitamin D resistant rickets: 1–3 μg/day.

1,25-dihydroxycholecalciferol

This is available for use in renal rickets. Dose is 1–3 μg/day. Regular monitoring of serum calcium essential.

Calcitonin

Mechanism

This lowers serum calcium by decreasing osteoclastic bone resorption and increasing renal calcium excretion.

Adverse effects

Nausea and flushing of the face are quite common. Inflammation can occur at injection site.

Clinical use and dose

Calcitonin is given by intramuscular or subcutaneous injection.
    Hypercalcaemia: 4–8 units/kg/day.
    Paget's disease of bone: 0.5–2 units/kg/day.
    These doses refer to synthetic porcine calcitonin. For longer term therapy the less immunogenic synthetic salmon calcitonin should be used.

Self poisoning

Self poisoning by drugs or other agents is a modern epidemic; it accounts for around 10% of acute medical admissions in the United Kingdom. Except in very young children, self poisoning is usually intentional.

Cases of intentional self poisoning may be divided into two groups:

(1) Those who genuinely attempt suicide; this group has a high incidence of depressive psychosis and schizophrenia.

(2) Those who use self poisoning to draw attention to their plight or to manipulate their social situation. Patients in this group often have inadequate personalities, often act impulsively and afterwards regret their action. Alcohol is involved in more than one-third of such cases.

It is clearly important in due course to make the distinction between the two in planning long-term management, but it has little relevance to immediate therapy.

21.1   GENERAL MANAGEMENT OF POISONING

Patients should be admitted to hospital, even if the degree of poisoning is trivial. This avoids an immediate repetition of the attempt and allows psychiatric evaluation once the drug effects have passed.

Initial assessment

History

Unless immediate cardiorespiratory resuscitation is required, the first thing to be done when the patient presents is to try and obtain an adequate relevant history. It is often necessary to question relatives or friends. Certain questions are of special importance:

(1) Has the patient actually taken an overdose? Patients have occasionally been treated on inadequate evidence, perhaps because a past history of drug abuse suggested this as the likely cause of an impaired conscious level.

(2) What drug or drugs were taken? Although most drugs require similar general supportive management, in some cases particular toxic effects can be anticipated, or enhancement of drug elimination might be appropriate.

(3) How much drug? This may matter less and estimates may be vague. Nevertheless, some guide to the potential seriousness of the problem is valuable in planning therapy. For example, 100 paracetamol tablets always cause serious toxicity; 10 nitrazepam tablets never do.

(4) Is the patient also taking other drugs, not necessarily in overdose, and is alcohol involved? For example, phenobarbitone, a hepatic enzyme inducer, worsens the hepatotoxicity caused by paracetamol. Alcohol obviously causes greater impairment of consciousness than might be expected from the dose of drug taken, and it may provoke hypothermia by vasodilatation.

(5) Is there a past history of impaired consciousness or convulsions? The patient may be in a post-ictal state.

(6) How was the drug obtained? This may appear of no immediate consequence, but the information may enable something to be done to help prevent another self-poisoning episode in future.

Clinical examination

A comprehensive clinical examination may well have to be deferred but particular attention should be paid at least to the following aspects:

Level of consciousness. This should not be described vaguely as 'drowsy' or 'comatose'. Coma is conventionally divided into four grades (Table 21.1). This is the minimum documentation required to permit assessment of the subsequent clinical course.

TABLE 21.1 Grades of coma

1. Drowsy but responds to vocal commands
2. Unconscious but responds to minimal stimuli
3. Unconscious and responds only to maximum painful stimuli
4. Unconscious and completely unresponsive

Drug-induced coma often has certain features which help in differentiation from other causes:

(1) Pupil reflexes are preserved, although this might be difficult to detect if the pupil is small.

(2) Reflex eye movements are absent. The two reflexes involved are doll's eye, in which rotation of the head produces contralateral deviation of the eyes, and the caloric reflex, in which instillation of cold water into the ear produces ipsilateral eye deviation.

Cardiovascular status. Hypotension is a common problem but serious elevations of blood pressure can also occur. Arrhythmias are common and tricyclic antidepressants may cause both tachycardia and heart block.

Respiratory status. Respiration can be compromised either by depression of the respiratory centre or aspiration into the lungs.

Temperature. Hypothermia below 35°C worsens the prognosis, especially in the elderly. If the axillary temperature is found to be low, the rectal temperature should be checked.

Evidence of other cause of impaired consciousness. Is there any evidence of head injury or are there localising neurological signs? Severe poisoning can sometimes cause false localising brainstem signs, but in general their presence raises the suspicion of another cause of coma.

Removal of ingested drug

An attempt should be made to prevent further drug from being absorbed, unless the risk from overdose is judged to be small.

Further absorption can be prevented in two ways:

(1) By recovering drug from the stomach,
(2) By adsorbing residual drug with medicinal charcoal.

Recovering drug from stomach

Unabsorbed drug can be removed from the stomach either by:
(1) Gastric lavage,
(2) Induced emesis.
This can be worthwhile 4–6 h after ingestion or even longer with agents such as aspirin or drugs with anticholinergic effects including tricyclic antidepressants and antihistamines, because these cause gastric atony.

Gastric lavage involves putting a wide-bore tube into the stomach and instilling warm water (500 ml). After a minute the water is removed and any tablet recovered retained for identification. The procedure may have to be repeated five or six times until no further drug is obtained. Care is required in the comatose patient. A suction tube should be applied to the pharynx to test for the presence of a gag reflex. If it is absent it is essential to have a cuffed endotracheal tube in place before gastric lavage is undertaken, thus avoiding aspiration. Gastric lavage can be traumatic. It must be undertaken with very great care if a corrosive poison has been taken and is contraindicated if petroleum distillate has been swallowed. The technique is impracticable in young children.

Induced emesis is effective, but less predictable, and its use is restricted to the conscious patient. It should not be used for corrosives or petroleum products. The agent used is Syrup of Ipecacuanha. This is safer than any other emetic agent. Emesis is usually produced within 20 min. If it is not, the dose can be repeated. Saline should not be used to induce emesis. It is not very effective and deaths have been caused by hypernatraemia when the risk of death without any treatment at all was very small.

Adsorbing drug

Effervescent activated charcoal (Medicoal) adsorbs residual drug, but 10 g of charcoal are needed to adsorb 1 g of drug. This limits its usefulness: for example, 10 g of charcoal adsorbs the equivalent of only two paracetamol tablets.

Continued management

With many drugs this amounts to support of the vital functions until the toxic effects of the drug have worn off.

Central nervous system

Convulsions can usually be controlled by intravenous chlormethiazole or diazepam. Convulsions that cannot be quickly brought under control by these means should be treated by muscle paralysis and ventilation since prolonged convulsions risk further brain damage.

Cardiovascular system

Tachyarrhythmias are treated conventionally, and heart block may require temporary transvenous cardiac pacing. Hypotension can often be corrected by raising the foot of the bed and giving intravenous fluids such as plasma or high molecular weight dextran.

The place of vasoconstrictor drugs is now controversial. Their use may compromise renal blood flow and other tissue perfusion. However, if the drug taken in overdose has caused vasodilatation, this can be reversed with metaraminol, 5 mg i.v. and this may be of value if intravenous fluids are contraindicated by cardiac failure.

Respiratory system

Modest respiratory depression can be treated with high concentrations of oxygen but more severe respiratory problems require ventilation.

Hypothermia

This should be corrected by wrapping the patient in foil to prevent further heat loss and by nursing in a warm atmosphere. If the patient is on a ventilator, warmed, humidified air is an effective method of raising the temperature.

It should be appreciated that optimal management requires the resources of an Intensive Therapy Unit, but provided such support is available an uncomplicated recovery can be expected in a great majority of cases of self poisoning.

Enhancing drug elimination

This is possible in only a minority of cases. It can alter the time course of recovery, but there is little evidence that the overall outcome is changed. Grade IV coma does carry a significant mortality, however, and in this case drug elimination should certainly be hastened to prevent complications such as hypostatic pneumonia and thromboembolic disease.

Forced alkaline diuresis (aspirin, phenobarbitone)

This can be employed only with drugs that are distributed mainly in the extracellular fluid and are largely excreted unchanged in the urine. The rationale is that the greater the proportion of drug in ionised form the less renal tubular reabsorption takes place, since only lipophilic un-ionised compounds readily cross cell membranes. Ionisation of acid drugs is encouraged by an alkaline medium. Accordingly, by rendering the urine alkaline, pH 7.5–8.5, more acid drug is excreted.

The technique of forced alkaline diuresis involves the administration of 1 litre of 5% dextrose and 500 ml of 1.2% sodium bicarbonate in the first hour with a further 1 litre dextrose and 500 ml bicarbonate over the next 3 h. Though this can be effective in increasing drug elimination three potential problem areas have to be monitored carefully:

(1) Precipitation of water intoxication and pulmonary or cerebral oedema, especially in the elderly. In that age group, central venous pressure should be measured. In general, if less than 350 ml urine in phenobarbitone poisoning, or less than 150 ml urine in aspirin poisoning is excreted in the first hour, 40 mg frusemide intravenously should be added.

Patients with aspirin poisoning are dehydrated initially.

(2) Serious alkalosis. Close monitoring of plasma pH is required. With aspirin the pH at presentation is variable. The drug ultimately causes acidosis, but this may be preceded by a respiratory alkalosis caused by hyperventilation.

(3) Hypokalaemia. The intracellular flux of potassium which accompanies this treatment causes hypokalaemia. 10–20 mmol potassium as potassium chloride may have to be added to each 500 ml of infusion fluid. Some authorities recommend doing this from the start, but it is probably best to adjust potassium supplementation in the light of continuing frequent serum electrolyte measurements.

Forced diuresis is not without hazard and should be reserved for moderate to severe toxicity. In the case of salicylates this means a plasma concentration above 3.5 mmol/l. However, it has recently been suggested that rendering the urine alkaline with sodium bicarbonate without additional fluid is at least as effective in enhancing aspirin excretion as the full forced diuretic regimen. This modification at least avoids the risk of fluid overload.

Forced acid diuresis, substituting arginine or lysine hydrochloride (10 g for 30 min) for the bicarbonate used in forced alkaline diuresis, is rarely employed. However, it may be helpful in quinine, amphetamine or fenfluramine overdosage.

Haemodialysis (lithium, severe alcohol poisoning)

Peritoneal dialysis is not advisable because peritoneal blood flow may be compromised in severely poisoned, hypotensive patients.

Haemodialysis is reserved for lithium (>3 mmol/l) and severe alcohol poisoning. When renal function is normal, it has no advantages over forced alkaline diuresis for salicylate and long-acting barbiturate poisoning.

Haemoperfusion (barbiturates, glutethimide, meprobamate, methaqualone, salicylates, chloral hydrate, theophylline.)

This technique involves the passage of blood through a column containing activated charcoal or resin onto which the drug is adsorbed. It is a major procedure requiring arterial and venous access. Formerly there was a risk of charcoal embolisation, thrombocytopenia and defibrination. Refinements to the columns, with the introduction of the resin amberlite, XAD-4, have improved matters. Haemorrhage, air embolism, infection and loss of a peripheral artery remain significant risks. It is undertaken only if the following criteria are satisfied:

The patient must:

(1) Be severely poisoned with Grade IV coma, major haemodynamic problems, respiratory depression or hypothermia,

(2) Be deteriorating clinically in spite of full resuscitative and supportive measures,

(3) Have developed complications such as pneumonia, septicaemia or shock lung,

(4) Have a high plasma drug level.

Even in these circumstances the technique is of value only if:
(1) The drug adsorbs onto charcoal or resin,
(2) A significant proportion of the drug is in the plasma compartment,
(3) Toxicity is related to the plasma level.

21.2 SPECIAL FEATURES OF CERTAIN DRUG OVERDOSE

Most cases of drug overdose can be managed by the conservative supportive measures discussed. A number of drugs deserve individual mention, however, because of particular clinical features or therapeutic measures warranted.

Barbiturates

It used to be thought that the formation of large skin blisters in overdosed patients was characteristic of barbiturates. It is now recognised that any coma may be responsible for their appearance in pressure areas. They are of no diagnostic value.

Medium-acting barbiturates, such as butobarbitone or amylobarbitone, are metabolised by the liver. In contrast with phenobarbitone toxicity, therefore, forced alkaline diuresis is of no value in treating overdose with these agents. Haemoperfusion is effective in severe poisoning.

Glutethimide

This may produce sudden apnoea secondary to raised intracranial pressure. The presence of raised intracranial pressure may be revealed by papilloedema which should be sought in poisoning with this drug. This sign may lag 48 h or more behind the development of raised pressure.

Urgent treatment is required with dexamethasone, 8 mg intravenously and 4 mg four times daily, supplemented with the osmotic diuretic, mannitol. 200 ml of the 20% mannitol solution is infused over 30 min. Although effective, mannitol must be administered with care in the elderly with monitoring of the central venous pressure to avoid the development of heart failure.

Antidepressant drugs

Monoamine oxidase inhibitors

These drugs prevent the breakdown of endogenous monoamines (Chapter 18.3), and this is the basis of the hypertension which is their most important toxic effect. Severe hypertension may result if a patient on a monoamine oxidase inhibitor takes food with a high content of sympathomimetic amines like tyramine. Overdose may present a complex picture including either hypertension or hypotension. The basis of the latter is not clear. Hyperreflexia and convulsions are also relatively common. Treatment is directed at the particular toxic effects which are prominent in individual patients.

Tricyclic antidepressants

These drugs inhibit noradrenaline reuptake in peripheral or central neurones, block parasympathetic muscarinic receptors and have a quindine-like effect on the heart (Chapter 18.3). Tachyarrhythmias may result. Alternatively, heart block and negative inotropic effects on the heart are also seen. Hypotension, especially orthostatic, is common. Ventricular fibrillation or other arrhythmias are not uncommon causes of death in tricyclic antidepressant poisoning. Electrocardiographic monitoring if possible in an Intensive Care Unit is indicated after more severe tricyclic overdoses. Agitation and convulsions also occur frequently. Several of these effects are due to parasympathetic blockade and this can be countered with a cholinesterase inhibitor (Chapter 19.4) by physostigmine (2 mg slow intravenous injection). Tachyarrhythmias may be controlled and the coma reversed quickly. The effect lasts for only about 20 min when the dose of physostigmine can be repeated. This is a relatively specific antidote but unless administered with great care it is easy to induce severe cholinergic effects.

Analgesics

Salicylates

Only in severe overdose does aspirin cause central nervous system depression. A severely poisoned patient may be alert, garrulous and even aggressive. It is easy to underestimate the severity of salicylate poisoning on clinical grounds. A metabolic acidosis caused by the drug itself may be complicated by a respiratory alkalosis induced by hyperventilation. Aspirin may still be recovered from the stomach 10 h after ingestion because of the gastric stasis induced by the drug. The efficacy of forced alkaline diuresis is such that the rate of aspirin excretion may be increased by a factor of twenty. It should be considered when plasma salicylate concentration is greater than 3.5 mmol/l and the patient is clinically toxic.

Opiates

Overdose is sometimes seen in drug addicts who, because of the variable potency of the preparations to which they have access, may accidentally take an overdose. The most powerful opiates such as morphine and diamorphine are seldom used in deliberate self-poisoning since they are usually administered parenterally. Penta-zocine is available in tablet form as is dextropropoxyphene. The latter has been widely prescribed in combination with paracetamol. In overdose this preparation may lead to profound respiratory depression caused by dextropropoxyphene and hepatotoxicity caused by paracetamol.

Opiates are unusual in having a specific and selective antagonist, naloxone (Chapter 17.2). This is a competitive antagonist, reversing their respiratory depressant effects and lacking itself any depressant effect on the respiratory centre. Naloxone 0.4 mg intravenously, repeated at 2–3 min intervals as required.

Paracetamol (Acetaminophen)

The main problem is hepatotoxicity. Paracetamol is metabolised by the liver. At therapeutic concentrations the major products are glucuronide and sulphate conjugates. A much smaller proportion is metabolised by the microsomal mixed function oxidases with the product of this pathway being detoxified by combination with glu-tathione. However, in overdose greatly increased amounts of para-cetamol are metabolised by this secondary pathway which exhausts glutathione stores and leaves an excess of a toxic metabolite. This then combines covalently with protein macromolecules in the liver to produce hepatic necrosis with a centrilobular pattern. If the patient survives, normal liver function is usually restored in a few months. The best guide to the likelihood of the development of hepatic necrosis is the plasma level of paracetamol and the rate of decline, the half-life, of the drug. A half-life of more than 4 h indicates saturation of the major routes of conjugation and potential toxicity. To wait for this information, however, requires a delay of more than 4 h from the patient's presentation before therapy is commenced. In practice, as a level of more than 1 mmol/l 4 h or more after ingestion suggests that hepatic necrosis is likely, treatment should be given. Fig. 21.1 gives a guide to management of paracetamol poisoning determined by plasma level and time after ingestion. To be effective, treatment must be begun as early as possible and certainly within 10 h of ingestion. It consists of either methionine given orally or N-acetyl cysteine given intravenously. Methionine enhances glutathione synthesis by the donation of thiol groups while N-acetyl cysteine is hydrolysed in vivo to cysteine, a glutathionine precursor. Thus, additional glutathione is made available to combine with the toxic metabolite and prevents binding to liver. In general oral methionine is the treatment of choice mainly because it is less than 5% the price of N-acetyl cysteine. However, the latter is useful in unconscious patients, such as those who take paracetamol in combination with dextropropoxyphene, or if vomiting is a problem.

Metal poisoning

Iron

The clinical presentation of iron poisoning may progress through three distinct phases:

(1) Iron is astringent and initially produces a gastritis, which may be erosive and haemorrhagic. It is seldom a serious problem, however, and the amount of blood loss is usually trivial. However, if vomiting and diarrhoea are severe they may lead to circulatory collapse.

(2) Even in severe untreated poisoning the initial gastritis usually resolves and the person's condition then appears satisfactory for

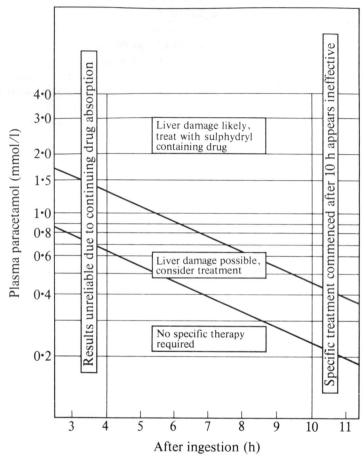

FIG. 21.1   Management of paracetamol poisoning.

12–24 h or even longer. This quiescent phase represents the interval between initial local astringent effects on the gastric mucosa and the toxic effects of absorbed iron. If the patient first presents during this phase it is vital not to be misled into assuming that no further problems will arise simply because gastritis and diarrhoea have resolved.

(3) If the natural course of the illness is not interrupted by treatment the third stage is entered about 24–48 h post-ingestion. It is

caused by widespread tissue poisoning by free iron, since the quantities absorbed following serious overdose may overwhelm the body's transfer and storage capacity. The prognosis is poor. Co-existing hepatic necrosis, cardiac and renal failure are further complicated by hypovolaemic shock resulting from a haemorrhagic enterocolitis. Central nervous system involvement follows with the onset of convulsions and then coma.

Desferrioxamine is a specific antidote for iron poisoning. It acts as a chelating agent for iron combining with it to form the octahedral complex ferrioxamine. It not only binds free iron but also removes it from transferrin and ferritin. The complex formed is excreted in the urine; so adequate renal function is necessary. Otherwise, haemodialysis to remove ferrioxamine is indicated.

At presentation, the patient is given desferrioxamine 2 g intramuscularly and gastric lavage is carried out, using 1 g for each lavage. 5 g is then left in the stomach to prevent absorption of any residual iron. Further desferrioxamine is then administered by slow intravenous infusion, not more than 15 mg/kg/h to a maximum of 80 mg/kg/h. A more rapid infusion may cause anaphylaxis and a larger total quantity itself produces renal damage. Treatment is continued until satisfactory serum iron concentrations (< 200 mmol/l) are reached or until transferrin is no longer 100% saturated. Desferrioxamine may be given by repeated intramuscular injection but this may cause pain at the injection site.

Other metals

Other chelating agents (d-penicillamine, dimercaprol and sodium calcium edetate) are useful in acute or chronic metal poisoning, particularly lead, copper or arsenic.

Comment

In 10% of cases, self poisoning requires intensive treatment; the remainder recover with simple nursing measures. Treatment in most cases is supportive. Gastric lavage or induced emesis are unnecessary when only a small amount of a relatively safe drug has been taken. There are only a few specific antidotes. Methods of increasing elimination carry their own risks and are effective with only a minority of drugs. They should, therefore, be reserved for cases of serious toxicity. Not every case requires detailed psychiatric evaluation but sympathetic management and appropriate social advice and help may avoid a recurrence.

CHAPTER 22

Use and misuse of common drugs

22.1   Adverse effects of 'over the counter' preparations

22.2   Drug interactions with 'over the counter' preparations

The desire to take medicine is one feature which distinguishes man, the animal, from his fellow creatures. It is really one of the most serious difficulties with which we have to contend.

Sir William Osler, 1894

A wide range of powerful pharmacological agents are easily available 'over the counter' from pharmacies or general retailers (Chapter 25). These pharmacy medicines or general sales list preparations are extensively used by the public. As they are often used without medical advice or direction, doctors may be unaware of the amount of such preparations being ingested.

In addition many patients do not view such preparations as real drugs and may omit to tell their doctor that they are taking them.

'Over the counter' preparations are of considerable importance because:

(1) They may cause adverse effects and toxicity leading to morbidity and, rarely, death.

(2) These preparations may interact with other drugs being given by a medical practitioner and cause adverse drug interactions.

319

22.1 ADVERSE EFFECTS OF 'OVER THE COUNTER' PREPARATIONS

Analgesics

Aspirin and other salicylates either alone, or in combination with agents such as caffeine and paracetamol, are commonly promoted for the relief of musculoskeletal aches and pains and headaches. While the former indication may be seen as an extension of the anti-inflammatory effect of prostaglandin synthesis inhibition (Chapter 11.2), the role of analgesic preparations in the treatment of non-specific recurrent tension headaches can be less well justified.

All aspirin-containing preparations carry a risk of increased gastrointestinal blood loss. This is usually chronic and occult, but may result in an acute haematemesis or melaena. Alcohol abuse increases the risk of bleeding and alcohol, by causing a 'hangover' headache, provides an excuse for self medication thus creating a vicious circle. Fortunately since the withdrawal of phenacetin from proprietary analgesics, chronic renal failure from interstitial nephritis and renal papillary necrosis is rare.

As aspirin and paracetamol are widely available in large amounts they are often used in self poisoning. Coma and hepatic necrosis respectively are consequences of overdose (Chapter 21.2).

Laxatives

Self purgation has been widely practised in the erroneous belief that a daily bowel action is essential for good health. Unfortunately the long-term use of powerful irritant purgatives such as senna leads to irreversible changes in colonic tone and severe constipation. Bulk laxatives such as bran are to be preferred if it is necessary to increase stool volume or frequency (Chapter 15.2).

Antacids

A wide range of alkali-containing preparations are available for symptomatic treatment of dyspepsia. Some contain anticholinergic drugs, which may cause adverse effects outside the intestine. Antacid preparations may cause either constipation or diarrhoea and excessive alkali intake, particularly with large amounts of milk may lead to hypercalcaemia, hypercalcuria and renal stone: the milk alkali syndrome.

Cold cures

While bacterial infections can be treated specifically with antibiotics there is no specific remedy for the common cold or other upper respiratory tract virus infections. A wide range of proprietary formulations offer a symptomatic relief of nasal congestion, rhinorhoea, pharyngitis and cough. These preparations may contain antihistamines (H_1-antagonists), sympathomimetics, simple analgesics and antitussive narcotic analogues.

Antihistamines may cause drowsiness and impairment of psychomotor function. Sympathomimetic drugs such as ephedrine or phenylpropanolamine may cause anxiety symptoms and tachycardia.

22.2 DRUG INTERACTIONS WITH 'OVER THE COUNTER' PREPARATIONS

Analgesics, purgatives, antacids and 'cold cures' may cause adverse drug interactions. As the 'over the counter' agent is usually taken without the physician's knowledge these interactions are not identified unless a careful drug history is taken. Antacids alter drug absorption either by binding the drug in an unabsorbable complex or by altering gastric emptying and small bowel transit time. Aspirin can compete for protein-binding sites displacing other drugs. In addition aspirin has direct effects on coagulation mechanisms and platelet functions and may potentiate the action of oral anticoagulants (Chapter 16.5).

Irritant purgatives may lead to hypokalaemia and increased digitalis toxicity (Chapter 6.6).

Ephedrine or phenylpropanolamine in 'cold cures' can provoke hypertension in patients receiving non-selective beta-blockers (Chapter 8.3). Similar agents may cause hypertensive crises in depressed patients treated with monoamine oxidase inhibitors (Chapter 18.3).

Comment

As the adverse effects and potential drug interactions after 'over the counter' preparations are clinically significant, remember the importance of an accurate drug history. Be aware that the patient may not consider an 'over the counter' preparation as a 'medicine'. Symptomatic relief by these preparations may obscure or disguise features of serious underlying pathology.

The patient's need for self-medication could be interpreted as a failure of communication on the part of the physician. Sympathetic attention, sound clinical judgement and counselling can reduce this unnecessary source of drug-related toxicity and misuse.

Development of new drugs

Aim

Drug development aims to produce a novel therapeutic agent which is superior in efficacy to existing remedies and which causes less frequent or less severe adverse effects.

23.1 EVOLUTION OF A NEW DRUG

The development of a new therapeutic agent involves a multidisciplinary group in many years of work. Formerly, drugs were extracted from natural plant and animal sources. Therapeutic use was empirical and based on traditional experience. Over the last 80 years an impressive number of drugs have been synthesised chemically. With the development of genetic engineering and the production of monoclonal antibodies it is likely that even more agents will be produced artificially.

Synthetic techniques have produced pure substances. This has led to increased specificity of action and, in some cases, greater efficacy and reduced toxicity. Unfortunately new drug development is expensive, and only a few substances (less than 1%) of those developed are actually marketed and used in practice.

The range of novel chemical entities developed has occasionally led to unexpected toxicity. As a consequence most governments have established bodies to regulate drug marketing, e.g. the *Committee on Safety of Medicines* in Britain, and the *Food and Drug Administration* in the United States. These agencies supervise clinical research on new drugs and licence new products. Although they serve to protect the public and are seen to do so, the statutory procedures that must be followed in applying for a licence for a new drug add greatly to the costs and time of development.

There is some evidence that the rate of introduction of entirely novel agents is slowing down. Whether this reflects economic pressures or diminished novel synthetic capacity or ability is not clear.

23.2 DRUG DEVELOPMENT STRATEGIES

Several strategies have been used in the development of new drugs. Over the years all have had success but no single approach has been consistently successful.

Serendipity, luck and intuition.

This approach has been applied less frequently in recent years. The discovery of penicillin by Fleming was in this category.

Molecular roulette.

Random chemical synthesis of new structures and pharmacological screening. This approach is wasteful and depends on the availability of sensitive animal or in vitro models of human disease, which often do not exist.

Minor structural changes in existing agents.

Occasionally this leads to compounds of greater efficacy and rarely to drugs with novel actions detected in pharmacological screening or clinical practice.

Programmed basic research with synthesis of specific chemical.

Intellectually this approach is the most satisfying. There have been spectacular results, e.g. levodopa and dopamine agonists in the treatment of Parkinsonism; beta-receptor blockers for angina; histamine (H_2) antagonists in peptic ulcer disease; converting enzyme inhibitors in hypertension. However, this approach is expensive and there is no guarantee of success.

Clinical observation of drug action in practice.

This is the traditional means of drug assessment. New applications arise from measurement of drug action in man in disease states. The antihypertensive effects of thiazide diuretics and beta-blockers were not predicted from animal screening tests. They were only identified after the drugs were available and were being used in practice.

23.3 EXPERIMENTAL PHARMACOLOGY

These studies determine whether the drug has the desired profile of action in model systems. The models are selected to provide as reliable an index of efficacy in man as possible.

Several models are usually employed. The models may be simple or complex and include:

(1) Cell cultures or bacteria,
(2) Partially purified enzymes or subcellular particles,
(3) Isolated tissues,
(4) Perfused organs,
(4) Intact animals from mice to primates.

The object is to identify therapeutically useful pharmacological activity and to characterise these actions using established models and drugs of known action.

When drugs with specific actions on enzymes or receptors are being studied, relatively simple cell free systems or isolated tissue preparations can be used. When poorly characterised subjective actions are sought, particularly involving behavioural effects, it may be necessary to perform tests in conscious intact animals.

23.4 TOXICOLOGICAL ASSESSMENT

In parallel with pharmacological experiments on efficacy, the toxic effects of acute and chronic dosing are determined. Acute toxicity is less important as long as LD_{50} (the dose that kills 50% of animals) is not close to the ED_{50} (the dose causing 50% of maximum pharmacological response).

Chronic toxicity testing is more relevant to clinical applications and should take place along the following lines:

(1) The route of administration, dose range, dose frequency and plasma levels should be appropriate to likely clinical indications. If possible, methods should be available to measure plasma concentrations and to determine patterns of metabolism.

(2) At least two species should be studied, usually dog and rat or mouse. If possible a species should be selected with a similar profile of metabolism to man.

(3) The duration of treatment should be consistent with the likely duration of use in man and the relative life expectancy of the animal species. Usually toxicity studies are undertaken over a period of 4 weeks to at least 1 year.

(4) Haematological and biochemical measurements should be made serially. All tissues should be examined histologically at death or on sacrifice of the experimental group. An untreated control group of littermates should be maintained for comparison.

Depending on the proposed patient group and disease indication, attention must be paid to:

(1) Effects on fertility in both males and females.

(2) Teratogenic effects on development of the embryo. The vulnerable period is very early in development, during organogenesis.

(3) Mutagenicity or an increased rate of mutation in germ cell lines or non-reproductive cells, e.g. bone marrow.

(4) Carcinogenicity or the induction or promotion of malignant tumours. There is disagreement over the relevance of some animal carcinogenicity studies to man.

Extensive formal toxicological tests are now required in most countries before drugs can be used on patients. There is considerable controversy as to the value of routine toxicology testing, as many differences between species, especially between man and rat, mouse, and dog, have been reported.

Paradoxically, thalidomide, which was the cause of the tragedy that led to stricter drug regulation and toxicology tests, is not teratogenic in mice or rats but has a teratogenic effect in humans, causing gross limb deformities.

23.5 CLINICAL EVALUATION

Only after animal studies have proved efficacy, and toxicological studies have provided a measure of the possible risk, can new drugs be given to humans. At this stage a further requirement is analytical evidence of chemical purity and pharmaceutical stability.

Evaluation in man can be considered in four phases. The relevance and extent of studies at these stages depends on the drug and its indications. Drugs for use in rare diseases, or in life-threatening and as yet untreatable states, may be evaluated in patient groups at an earlier stage than those with readily measurable effects on common diseases.

Phase 1 involves small scale studies in normal volunteers. These studies should determine whether the drug can be given to man without serious symptoms or toxicity, and whether it has the desired pharmacological effects. These studies often begin with a dose-ranging study, using 1/50 to 1/100 the effective dose in animals and increasing until the desired effect, or adverse effects, are seen. These studies should only be performed on volunteers who are informed about the implications of the tests, and who give their consent freely. Studies should include careful assessment of clinical, haematological and biochemical evidence before and after drug administration to identify pharmacological actions and adverse effects. Phase 1 studies should only be performed by experienced staff, under medical supervision, and in premises with appropriate resuscitative facilities and support.

Phase 2 studies determine whether the new drug has the desired effect on patients with the appropriate disease. In Britain these investigations can be performed only after submission of preclinical and Phase 1 study results to the *Committee on Safety of Medicines*. This body either issues a clinical trial certificate (CTC) or authorises limited clinical trials under an exemption procedure (CTE). Phase 2 studies initially may be open, uncontrolled, dose-ranging experiments but should include controlled studies under single or double-blind conditions. They may involve comparisons with inactive placebo or known active agents.

Phase 3. If results of therapeutic efficacy and safety justify it, the next step is progression to large scale clinical trials to determine how the new drug compares in clinical practice with existing remedies, and to establish its profile of action and frequency of adverse effects.

After Phase 3 studies the evidence from all stages of development is assembled and if the conclusions indicate a useful action, the drug may be submitted to the regulatory authorities with a request for a product licence.

Phase 4. A new drug is usually marketed after only a few hundred, or at the most a few thousand, patients have been exposed to it for a relatively short period (weeks or months). As discussed in Chapter 24, post-marketing surveillance is increasingly undertaken to assess efficacy and toxicity of new drugs on a larger scale. No uniform scheme for Phase 4 supervision has yet been established, but few doubt the necessity of collecting this information on low-frequency adverse effects.

23.6 MARKETING AND PROMOTION

The rationale for the development of new drugs should be to provide better drugs; better in the sense of being either more effective, safer or cheaper. Unfortunately, only a small proportion of 'new' drugs actually represent a truly novel development or application. More often, 'new' drugs at best incorporate modest molecular variations based on existing drugs, or pharmaceutical formulation changes which have a marginal effect on absorption, toxicity or efficacy. At worst they are copies of existing drugs or minor reformulations to extend patent rights and royalties.

Drug development is expensive. This is borne by the pharmaceutical industry, which justifiably expects to recoup the cost of development when the product is finally marketed. In some therapeutic areas where drugs are widely used, e.g. antibiotics, nonsteroidal anti-inflammatory drugs, analgesics, antihypertensives, heavy investment in marketing and promotion has led to the use of undistinguished new drugs in place of equally effective, cheaper and established alternatives whose side effect profile is well known. Therapeutic fads and fashions should be avoided and prescribing practices changed only when good evidence of improved efficacy or reduced toxicity is available.

The physician needs guidance on critical assessment of what represents an important advance. Unfortunately, his most accessible source of information is the representative of the pharmaceutical manufacturer who has been specially trained and briefed to promote his particular new product; indeed his livelihood depends on the ability to do so.

Practitioners must seek out alternative sources of information from district or regional information pharmacists, specialist clinical colleagues, postgraduate meetings and publications in the scientific literature. Publications, in themselves, can be misleading. Evidence from a few controlled studies published in well established journals subject to peer review are more reliable than bulky obscure proceedings of sponsored meetings to promote a particular drug.

Physicians should make an active attempt to determine in what way a new drug represents an improvement over existing therapy, and what is the price in terms of adverse effects and actual cost of the drug.

As new drugs may be marketed after studies in only a few hundred or thousand patients, special vigilance is required in the first few years of use to determine low frequency, but potentially serious adverse effects.

Comments

New drug developments should be examined critically; objective evidence from several sources should be sought to highlight improved therapeutic efficacy and reduced toxicity in controlled comparison with established remedies.

CHAPTER 24

Adverse drug reactions

24.1 DEFINITION AND MAGNITUDE OF THE PROBLEM

An adverse drug reaction can be defined as 'any undesired or unintended effect of drug treatment'. This definition is intentionally very broad and includes such effects as an acute allergic reaction to penicillin, severe hypoglycaemia after excessive insulin administration, osteoporosis after long-term corticosteroid therapy, rebound hypertension after discontinuing clonidine and phocomelia in the children of mothers exposed to thalidomide during early pregnancy.

It has been estimated that an average hospital medical patient receives between five and ten different drugs during a 10 day stay in hospital. During this time about 25% of patients experience one or more adverse drug effects, and 1% experience a life-threatening event due to drugs. Of these the majority are patients who have tumours and develop pancytopenia as a result of cancer chemotherapy. Only one in a thousand medical patients suffers a life-threatening adverse drug effect in which the risks of therapy seemed in retrospect to outweigh the potential benefits. The potential for

TABLE 24.1 Adverse drug effects

Predictable reactions
Excess pharmacological activity.
Rebound response upon discontinuation.

Unpredictable reactions
Allergic effects.
Genetically-determined effects.
Idiosyncratic effects.

adverse reaction is even greater in general practice. Some 25% of acute medical admissions to hospital can be attributed in whole or in part to the adverse effects of drug therapy.

Older age groups receive a disproportionately high number of prescriptions for drugs and adverse drug reactions are particularly common in this group for pharmacokinetic, pharmacodynamic and social reasons.

Adverse drug effects can be classified in many ways. A useful approach to the problem is given in Table 24.1. In this scheme adverse effects are grouped into those that are predictable on the basis of the drugs known actions and those that are not. The former type usually occurs early in the course of treatment, is a common event which is dose related and is either recognised as a possibility before clinical trials begin or very shortly thereafter. By contrast, the latter type is usually infrequent, rarely recognised until widespread use of the medicine has occurred and need not necessarily be dose dependent.

24.2 PREDICTABLE ADVERSE REACTIONS

Excessive pharmacological effects

Predictable adverse drug effects are due to excessive pharmacological activity of the drug in question. This arises particularly with central nervous system depressants, cardioactive, hypotensive and hypoglycaemic agents. Specific examples of this type of reaction are:

(1) Respiratory depression in severe bronchitic patients given morphine or benzodiazepine hypnotics.

(2) Hypotension resulting in stroke, myocardial infarction or renal failure in patients receiving excessive doses of antihypertensive drugs.

(3) Bradycardia in patients receiving excessive digoxin.

Less obvious but equally important are predictable adverse effects where the particular pharmacological effect involved is not the one for which the drug was initially administered. For example, a patient receiving an antihistamine for the prevention of motion sickness may become drowsy.

All patients are at risk of developing this type of reaction if high doses are given. However, certain subgroups are particularly susceptible (Chapters 2 and 3) and include those with renal disease, liver disease, the very young and the elderly.

Withdrawal symptoms or rebound responses after discontinuation of treatment

This type of reaction is unusual in that it occurs in the absence of the causative agent. The abrupt interruption of therapy is followed by a characteristic withdrawal syndrome:

(1) Extreme agitation, tachycardia, confusion, delirium and convulsions may occur following discontinuation of long-term central nervous system depressants such as barbiturates, benzodiazepines and alcohol.

(2) Acute Addisonian crisis may be precipitated by abrupt cessation of corticosteroid therapy.

(3) Severe hypertension and symptoms of sympathetic overactivity may arise shortly after discontinuing clonidine therapy.

(4) Withdrawal symptoms after narcotic analgesics.

In all these instances adaptation has occurred to the drug at the receptor level. This adaptation is usually associated with some tolerance to the effects of the drug, and a gradually increasing dose of drug may be necessary to sustain the initial effect. Withdrawal effects may be minimised by gradual withdrawal of the drugs involved or by substitution with longer-acting or less potent agents and gradual withdrawal.

24.3   UNPREDICTABLE ADVERSE EFFECTS

Allergic drug responses

Drug *allergy* or hypersensitivity are common adverse drug effects. Indeed some clinicians regard this type of response as being the single most frequent adverse drug effect. Such reactions are unpredictable and are often not dose related. They occur only in a small proportion of the population exposed to the drug, and it is usually impossible to predict the response in advance. These reactions vary from mild erythematous skin reactions to major anaphylactic shock. An allergic adverse effect of a drug is characterised by the fact that:

(1) The reaction does not resemble the expected pharmacological effect of the drug.

(2) There is delay between first exposure to the drug and the development of a reaction.

(3) The reaction recurs upon repeated exposure even to traces of the drug.

The drugs most frequently associated with allergic skin reactions are the penicillins, the sulphonamides and blood products.

Genetically-determined effects

The major toxicity of some drugs is restricted to individuals with a particular genotype or genetic make-up. Thus patients with hereditary pseudocholinesterase deficiency are unable to metabolise the muscle relaxant succinyl choline and may develop prolonged paralysis and apnoea following its use (Chapter 17.5). Similarly, individuals with glucose-6-phosphate dehydrogenase deficiency are at substantial risk of developing acute haemolytic anaemia after exposure to the antimalarial drug primaquine and to sulphonamides and quinidine. Some of the most common types of genetic abnormalities that may lead to drug toxicity are shown in Table 24.2.

Genetically-determined acetylator polymorphism affects responses and adverse effects to isoniazid, hydralazine and procainamide. Such drugs are metabolised in the liver by the enzyme N-acetyl

TABLE 24.2 Some genetically-determined types of drug toxicity

Pseudocholinesterase deficiency.	Succinylcholine.	Paralysis, apnoea
Glucose-6-phosphate dehydrogenase deficiency.	Sulphonamides, Quinidine, Primaquine.	Haemolysis.
Acetylator polymorphism.	Procainamide, Hydralazine, Isoniazid.	Systemic lupus (in slow acetylators), Neuropathy (in slow acetylators).
Hepatic porphyria.	Barbiturates.	Symptomatic porphyria.

transferase. There is a bimodal distribution of acetylator capacity in the population, with some individuals being *slow* and others *fast* acetylators (Chapter 1). Slow acetylators of isoniazid given standard doses are much more likely to suffer from perpiheral neuropathy than fast acetylators. The drug-induced lupus syndrome is much more common in slow acetylators receiving hydralazine or procainamide. Adverse effects of hydralazine and also gold salts and d-penicillamine are linked to the specific histocompatibility antigens. In the future, tissue typing may help to predict susceptibility to drug toxicity.

Idiosyncratic drug reactions

The term *idiosyncrasy* is used primarily to cover unusual, unexpected or bizarre drug effects that cannot readily be explained or predicted in individual recipients. Also included in this type of reaction are drug-induced fetal abnormalities such as phocomelia (limb deformity), which developed in the offspring of mothers receiving thalidomide in early pregnancy.

Drug-induced malignant disease is fortunately rare and may be considered an idiosyncratic drug effect:

(1) Analgesic abuse may rarely cause cancer of the renal pelvis.

(2) Long-term oestrogens without coincidental progestogens may induce uterine cancer.

(3) Immunosuppressive drugs may induce lymphoid tumours.

(4) Intramuscular iron preparations may cause sarcomata at the site of injection.

(5) Thyroid cancer may develop in patients who have received ^{131}I-therapy in the past.

24.4 DISCOVERY OF DRUG-INDUCED DISEASE

Before a new drug is released for widespread use the manufacturer must obtain a licence from the appropriate government authority (*Committee on Safety of Medicines* in U.K., *Food and Drug Administration* in U.S.A., *Department of Drugs* in Sweden, etc.) (Chapter 23). It is likely that over 3000 healthy volunteers and patients will have received the drug in supervised trials before permission for general marketing is given, unless the drug is for a rare disease when experience may be much smaller. By this stage most of the pharmacological effects are known. Adverse effects resulting from excess pharmacological activity may be well documented. This is, however, not the case for unpredictable toxicity. Such adverse effects are often not identified until it has been subjected to much more widespread use. Only after several years was it recognised that the beta-receptor blocking drug practolol could cause an oculomucocutaneous syndrome when taken regularly over a long period. Likewise, thalidomide had been marketed for several years before its potential for causing severe limb deformities (phocomelia) in the offspring of mothers taking it in early pregnancy was appreciated.

In order to identify unexpected adverse drug effects several different approaches have been adopted.

Cohort study

This is used when groups of drug recipients are followed to evaluate outcomes after drug exposure.

Spontaneous report of suspected adverse drug reactions

This occurs when prescribers report suspected reactions to a central agency which investigates, collates and reviews the resulting information.

Review of vital statistics

This occurs when epidemiologists review national or regional statistics to note any unusual epidemics of diseases or uncommon disorders.

Case-control study

This is used when patients with suspected drug-induced disease are compared with a reference population.

Each approach has its strengths and weaknesses but the different types of study are complimentary.

Cohort studies

These generally allow the detection of events occurring with a frequency of greater than 1 per 500 exposed. Various types of cohort study have been conducted to detect drug toxicity.

Short-term clinical trials are expensive to conduct and time consuming. They are usually done early in the life-time of a drug and are confined to patients who have no disorders other than those relevant to the drug in question. Thus the approach is useful only in detecting and quantitating common acute adverse drug effects.

Long-term clinical trials are formidable undertakings and are rarely conducted. They are expensive to organise and maintain. They are confined to medications which are used on a long-term basis, e.g. oral contraceptives, antidiabetic drugs and antihypertensive drugs. When successful they give useful information both on acute and delayed effects of drug treatment. However, there are often problems in maintaining the integrity of the study cohort and in demonstrating that satisfactory randomisation of the treated and control groups has been carried out.

Post-marketing surveillance of established drugs. Studies in which a group of recipients is identified and observed for possible adverse effects are now being conducted more frequently. The periods of observation are usually brief (days or weeks) and the size of the cohorts small (rarely more than 2000). Such studies are useful for quantifying known acute effects after short-term exposure to drugs and for identifying subgroups of the population who are at greatest risk of toxicity, e.g. elderly, those with renal impairment, liver disease, etc.

Post-marketing surveillance of new drugs. This approach is relatively new. It aims to review a large cohort of 10 000 or more recipients of a drug newly released onto the market and to follow such individuals for a substantial period: at least one and preferably several years. If successful, such studies have the potential for detecting both acute and delayed toxicity following short- or long-term exposure. Once again a major problem is to maintain the integrity of the study cohort. Although less expensive to conduct than a long-term clinical trial, such studies are nevertheless likely to be confined to those new drugs that are used for prolonged periods in large numbers of patients.

These studies give not only an indication of what reactions may occur but also some idea of the frequency with which they may be expected.

Spontaneous reports of suspected adverse drug reactions

In USA, UK, Scandinavia and most western European countries there are agencies that collect information about suspected adverse drug effects. For example, in the UK, the *Committee on Safety of Medicines* has an adverse reaction sub-committee, which encourages physicians to report suspected adverse drug reaction on a standard form. The resulting information is analysed regularly to determine whether or not any unusual patterns of reports are emerging. Unfortunately it has a relatively low response rate, particularly from hospital-based physicians. It has not been successful in detecting previously unsuspected reactions to drugs.

Not surprisingly if a reaction is unsuspected, the doctor's index of suspicion is low. Spontaneous reporting has been useful, however, in confirming whether or not a newly suspected reaction is widespread in the community. This approach, however, only assesses the number of suspected reactions. There is no estimate of the frequency of reactions because it gives no details of the numbers exposed to the drug in the population from which the reports were received.

Vital statistics

A review of national or regional health-care statistics should be in theory a useful way of detecting an unsuspected epidemic of an unusual condition or a marked increase in prevalence of a common condition. This might prove to be so if the collection of such statistics were sufficiently accurate and data processing and review undertaken sufficiently rapidly. At present this approach is not practical. In the West of the USA an epidemic of uterine cancer occurred during the 1970s. This was well documented in the regional statistics but no-one appreciated its significance until isolated reports linking long-term oestrogen use to uterine cancer were published. By then the major epidemic was already under way. Efficient and informed review of the vital statistics could well have led to the discovery of this problem 2 or 3 years earlier. Regular perusal of accurate regional vital statistics could indicate conditions which showed an unexpected increase and therefore might be drug induced.

Case-control studies

The drug consuming habits of patients with a suspected drug-induced disease are compared with those of a reference population who do not have the suspect disease. This approach is increasingly being used to detect and quantify drug-related disease. It is particularly useful in showing associations between drug use and rare diseases where the risks of developing the disease are less than 1 in 500 persons exposed. Under those circumstances, it would be prohibitively expensive and complex to attempt to follow a cohort of recipients, and it is easier to start at the suspected disease and work back to the drug exposure.

In case-control studies the results are expressed as *relative risks*: that is, for example, the risk of being a cigarette smoker in a series of patients with lung cancer compared to the risk in reference patients without lung cancer. This information is insufficient to assess the actual risk of getting lung cancer if one is a smoker. Calculating such a risk requires additional information not usually available to those conducting the case-control study.

There are major limitations to case-control studies.

(1) While they may show associations between diseases and drug use, they do not prove that these associations are causal.

(2) They are difficult to conduct in practice since they can be subject to bias either as a result of the type of reference population studied or of foreknowledge of the hypothesis under review by the interviewer.

(3) It is important to confine interest to newly diagnosed cases in order to avoid distortion of drug-consuming habits as a consequence of awareness of the presence of a significant disease. For example: when assessing the association between chronic renal failure and analgesic abuse, it would not be advisable to look at previously diagnosed cases of renal failure since such patients are likely to have been advised to avoid drugs in general and analgesics in particular. A case-control study which included previously diagnosed cases of renal failure amongst the cases could therefore produce a result which did not show any drug association with analgesic abuse even if, in reality, analgesic abuse was indeed associated with significant risk of chronic renal failure.

Using these techniques it is likely that the ability to detect serious drug-related toxicity will greatly improve in the 1980s. Provided these limitations are appreciated and the resulting information is handled efficiently, this approach has much to offer particularly when we are dealing with rare or delayed drug effects.

24.5 REDUCTION OF THE RISK OF ADVERSE EFFECTS

Many powerful drugs are now available. It is hardly surprising that occasionally untoward effects are produced. With better knowledge of the pharmacological mechanisms whereby drugs exert their effects, and their toxicity, and the pathophysiology of diseases, it is likely that in the future drug therapy may become safer. The risks of developing adverse drug effects can be reduced by observing simple rules:

(1) Always include a detailed drug history as part of clinical history or consultation

(2) Only use drug treatment when there is a clear indication for it and there is no non-pharmacological alternative

(3) Avoid multiple drug regimens and combination tablets whenever possible

(4) Pay particular attention to drug dose and response in:
the young, the old and those with coexisting renal, hepatic or cardiac disease.

(5) Review the need for continuing treatment regularly and stop drugs which are no longer necessary.

CHAPTER 25

Drug prescription:
legal and practical aspects

25.1 Legal aspects of prescribing in the United Kingdom

25.2 Practical aspects of prescribing

> *Man may escape from rope and gun;*
> *nay, some have out-liv'd the doctor's pill*
>
> John Gay (1685–1732)

Although a medicine and its active drug constituents can have a powerful effect in the treatment of disease and the alleviation of symptoms, the inappropriate choice of drug or the incorrect dose of an appropriate drug could lead to serious morbidity or even mortality. The choice of therapeutic agent must be based on information gained from clinical history, examination and any necessary further investigations. Other factors that influence the choice are the age of the patient and associated pathology (renal or hepatic disease).

Once the decision has been made, the patient must be supplied with the medicine or treatment. The importance of this stage has often been ignored both in practice and in the training of doctors. Poor communication by the medical practitioner is a major factor in poor compliance of the patient with instructions (Chapter 26). Clear, unambiguous instructions to the patient are essential not only to indicate the dose and frequency with which the medicine is to be taken but also to reinforce any additional advice about diet, smoking and the level of social and physical activity.

In most countries there are restrictions on the availability of drugs. In the United Kingdom medicines are classified into three categories.

(1) *General sales list preparations* are medicines that can be supplied by most retailers in supermarkets, etc. Some simple analgesics, e.g. aspirin, and antacids are widely available for sale. These preparations may be used excessively or inappropriately and can contribute to drug-related morbidity either by direct toxicity or through drug interactions (Chapter 22).

(2) *Pharmacy medicines*, which may only be supplied by a registered pharmacist, may be supplied to a patient without a prescription from a registered medical practitioner. These 'over the counter' preparations may cause adverse effects and interact with other prescribed drugs (Chapter 22).

(3) *Prescription-only medicines* can only be supplied by a pharmacist on the prescription of a registered medical (or dental) practitioner.

Comment

Details of legal requirements vary in different countries. The ethical and practical responsibilities are universal.

25.1 LEGAL ASPECTS OF PRESCRIBING IN THE UNITED KINGDOM

Prescribing of drugs in the United Kingdom is regulated by the *Medicines Act of 1968*, the *Misuse of Drugs Act of 1971* and the *Misuse of Drugs Regulations of 1973*.

Controlled drugs

Under the *Misuse of Drugs Regulations of 1973*, drugs with a high abuse potential, drugs of addiction and other drugs with non-therapeutic psychotropic activity are categorised as *controlled drugs*. These drugs, which include narcotic analgesics, cocaine, barbiturates, amphetamines and related agents, can only be prescribed by registered medical practitioners. Controlled drugs are divided into four *schedules*, only two of which are therapeutically relevant:

Schedule I includes weak narcotic analgesics and dilute preparations of morphine, such as mixture of kaolin and morphine BP used for symptomatic treatment of diarrhoea.

Schedule II includes morphine, heroin, other narcotics, cocaine and amphetamines.

Prescriptions for Schedule II controlled drugs must follow specified legal guidelines:

(1) The prescription must be written in the physician's own handwriting.

(2) The prescription must include the name and address of the patient.

(3) The medicine or drug, the dose and the quantity to be supplied or the total number of doses should be stated in figures and words, e.g. 10 (ten) mg.

(4) The prescription must be signed and dated by the practitioner and include his address.

The requirements for controlled drug prescription are the basis of good prescription writing and should be used as a model for *all* prescriptions.

There are legal obligations on medical practitioners to report to the Home Office for registration any patient who is believed to be dependent or addicted to controlled drugs. The legal aspects of drug regulation and the control of drug abuse are further reviewed in the *British National Formulary*.

25.2 PRACTICAL ASPECTS OF PRESCRIBING

It is obvious that while appropriate drug therapy can be of great benefit, inappropriate therapy is not harmless. On all occasions, there should be a positive reason for prescribing a drug. Drug treatment should never become a routine. In hospital it is still not uncommon to find 'routine' prescriptions for hypnotics, analgesics and purgatives without any consideration of individual need. Many patients and doctors expect a consultation to result automatically in prescription of a medicine. Both of these procedures are undesirable and bad prescribing practice.

When drug treatment is indicated, it is mandatory that the most appropriate agent is given in the correct dose and in a regimen which results in optimum treatment with minimum adverse effects.

When the treatment has been selected, the doctor communicates his wishes to the pharmacist and the patient by his prescription. Accurate communication with the pharmacist is essential if the patient is to receive the desired treatment.

Prescriptions for medicines should be written legibly either typewritten or ink (mandatory for controlled drugs) and clearly in English. There is no justification for writing illegible or unintelligible prescriptions. The use of Latin or Greek terms or obscure abbreviations is anachronistic and liable to be misunderstood by nursing staff and/or patients.

(1) Specify the patient's full name, address and age.

(2) Indicate clearly the drug or medicine. As discussed below it is preferable to use the approved or generic name rather than the proprietary or brand name.

(3) Specify precisely the strength of tablets, capsules or mixtures. It is good prescribing practice to indicate these in words and figures and mandatory for prescriptions of controlled drugs.

(4) Indicate the dose frequency and total quantity to be supplied or the duration of treatment. Once again it is good practice to include these in words and figures as this is a legal requirement for controlled drugs.

(5) Do not leave large blank spaces on the prescription, which may be filled in by forgery to obtain unauthorised supplies of abused drugs.

(6) Sign the prescription, date it and indicate your name and address. Addition of a telephone number assists the pharmacist in contacting the prescriber in the case of a prescription for an unusual drug or dose regimen.

Approved (generic) or proprietary (brand) name prescribing?

Drugs available on prescription have approved or generic names. Individual manufacturers give their own preparations proprietary (brand or trade) names. A drug that is not covered by patent rights may be available in several proprietary formulations of the same generic preparation. There are obvious commercial pressures to encourage proprietary prescription. Proprietary names are usually short, snappy and memorable. They do not, however, necessarily give any indication of the active ingredients of the medicine. All marketed preparations have passed basic standards of purity and safety. They may differ in their formulation and this may affect absorption and distribution. Although there have been a few examples where formulation differences have led to marked changes in effect and toxicity, on the vast majority of occasions the minor pharmaceutical differences between formulations are irrelevant in clinical practice. It is good prescribing practice to use the generic name of drugs unless there is a very compelling reason for using brand names, for example, when a combination tablet is being used. In Britain proprietary prescription in general practice legally compels the pharmacist to provide that particular brand with attendant inconvenience to the pharmacist and often delay to the patient. As proprietary preparations vary greatly in price, generic prescribing may result in a prescription of a less expensive preparation with attendant savings in the overall cost of drug treatment. Comparative costs of *equivalent* preparations can be readily asssessed from the *British National Formulary*.

The *British National Formulary* is published by the British Medical Assocation and the Pharmaceutical Society of Great Britain twice a year and is provided free to practising doctors and medical students in the United Kingdom. All marketed medicines are listed systematically together with brief notes on adverse effects, contra-indications and details of dosage. It is a practical pocket reference manual. It should be used in conjunction with textbooks and monographs which provide background information on the rational basis of treatment and guidance on the choice of drug from a list of preparations.

Good prescribing practice

(1) Familiarise yourself with a *limited* number of well-established drugs with *known* effects and side-effects. Do *not* chop and change amongst equivalent preparations on whim or fancy. Avoid trying out new preparations simply because of novelty or extensive commercial promotion. Always prescribe by generic or approved names.

(2) Try to devise a treatment regimen which allows drugs to be given once or twice daily. Try to reduce the total number of drugs being given to a minimum and encourage patients to take medicines at a convenient time or place in their daily routine. Avoid vague terms like 'with food' or 'after meals' as the frequency of

drug taking may depend on the number of meals taken each day. However, if it is intended that a medicine, such as a non-steroidal anti-inflammatory drug, is taken with food, then state this and the frequency. Always avoid the use of 'as before' or 'as directed' and specify the dose and frequency. Do not prescribe 'as required' without stating the maximum dose and dose interval.

(3) Check the dose carefully each time you prescribe. Do not trust to memory and be particularly careful when doses are in the microgram range or when prescribing for children and the elderly.

(4) It is now routine practice in Britain to indicate to the patient on his prescription the name of the medicine. Avoid labels like 'the tablets' or 'the mixture'. Of course, on rare occasions such as the use of narcotic or cytotoxic drugs in patients with cancer it may be justifiable to withhold the proper name.

(5) Use compound preparations and combination tablets only when there is an established therapeutic need for all the constituents, and where the combination of two or more drugs aids compliance.

(6) Finally, always review drug prescriptions regularly: every day in hospital patients or weekly or monthly as appropriate in out-patients or general practice. When reviewing prescriptions ask the questions:

  (a) Is the drug treatment still necessary?
  (b) Is the optimum dose regimen being followed?
  (c) Is the desired effect being achieved?
  (d) Are there any symptoms or adverse effects which could be secondary to drug treatment?

Do not continue treatment by repeating prescriptions over long periods of time without assessing the response in the patient, or worse still, without seeing the patient.

Comment

The basis of good prescribing is a sound training in clinical methods and pathophysiology, which together with an understanding of pharmacodynamic and pharmacokinetic properties of the drugs being used, permits maximum benefit to be achieved with the minimum risk of adverse effects. Prescriptions are legal documents. They should consist of clear, legible instructions to the pharmacist. Illegible, incomplete or ambiguous prescriptions are not only bad medicine, they are illegal.

CHAPTER 26

Compliance with drug therapy

26.1 Size of the problem

26.2 Detection of poor compliance

26.3 Improving compliance

It is an ironical fact of modern medicine that despite tremendous advances in diagnostic *accuracy*, if the patient fails to take the recommended treatment, the expense and effort involved are virtually wasted. It is implicit in all prescribing that the patient takes the treatment as directed, yet there is overwhelming evidence that this is simply not the case. Indeed, in certain conditions, the majority of patients do not take their medication appropriately. This is called *non-compliance*.

26.1 SIZE OF THE PROBLEM

Approximately one-third of out-patients take their treatment as directed, one-third partly comply and one-third never comply. Poor compliance is found in all socio-economic and racial groups and there is no satisfactory method of predicting who will fail to comply with treatment. However, it is known that compliance is likely to be decreased in certain circumstances:

(1) The very young and the very old.

(2) Patients requiring long-term treatment.

(a) Conditions that are asymptomatic but which require long-term therapy: hypertension is the classical example. Some studies have shown that 6 months after starting treatment for hypertension as many as 50% of patients are failing to comply.

(b) Conditions where the patient has some psychiatric disease such a psychosis.

(3) Failure to understand that treatment is beneficial or that the disease is potentially dangerous.

(4) Complexity of treatment. Prescription of too many drugs in different doses. Difficulty of access to the drugs, for example, when a patient with rheumatoid arthritis is faced with a child-proof container.

(5) Adverse effects: though if these are genuinely unavoidable they might be tolerated if the treatment is seen to be beneficial.

(6) Expense: this is likely to be a factor in those countries where medicines are purchased at their full value. However, it must be recognised that the provision of drugs at no or very low cost, for example by the National Health Service in the UK, does not greatly influence compliance.

26.2 DETECTION OF POOR COMPLIANCE

This is not easy. Doctors in general believe that poor compliance happens to *other* doctors' patients. There are, however, certain simple procedures which can help in detecting poor compliance.

Ask the patient how he or she is getting on with the medication and whether they are finding it easy to take the treatment as prescribed. A friendly enquiry of this nature might reveal poor compliance and the reasons for it.

Assessment of pharmacological effect. This is clearly easier for some drugs than for others. A patient receiving a beta-blocker, for example, should have a relative bradycardia. In general terms failure to achieve a therapeutic goal should always raise the question of poor compliance.

Assessment of the rate of drug consumption. This has its limitations as medication can be disposed of easily, but two approaches can be tried. In general practice the actual and expected rate at which repeat prescriptions are requested might show a gross disparity, suggesting that the medication is not being taken at the expected rate. The other approach is to count the number of tablets in the drug container and to calculate the number used since the last clinic visit. The patient must bring the medication to the doctor and this has the additional advantage that the patient can be asked to identify a use for each drug. Genuine misunderstanding which might have led to inappropriate drug taking can be corrected. Diazepam taken each morning to control atrial fibrillation with a digoxin tablet occasionally at night to help the patient sleep might not be what the doctor had in mind!

Drug level monitoring is becoming increasingly available (Chapter 5). Its most definitive role in determining compliance is the finding of unexpectedly low levels or no drug at all in the plasma. Levels that are merely sub-therapeutic might be the result of poor compliance but could also reflect abnormally low bioavailability or high clearance. Quantitative assessment can be made of many drugs in saliva. As a simple screening manoeuvre it may be useful to perform qualitative tests for the presence or absence of drugs in urine.

26.3 IMPROVING COMPLIANCE

There is no absolutely reliable method of ensuring compliance with drug therapy. However, the following may be helpful:

Patient counselling. Explain clearly to the patient, or relatives where appropriate, why treatment is necessary and what is likely to be achieved by the treatment.

Keep treatment regimen simple. Wherever possible use once or twice daily doses and try to avoid the need for a mid-day dose. Review drug treatment regularly to assess whether *all* treatment is *still* necessary.

Treatment schedule. Explain when the drugs should be taken and in what dose. In addition to explaining verbally write it down as the patient may forget your instructions.

Various attempts are being made by the pharmaceutical industry to improve compliance by the use of aids such as calendar packs and treatment diaries. Although attractive in theory there is currently no evidence that these actually improve patient compliance.

Outline possible adverse effects and encourage the patient to contact you before the next appointment if symptoms get worse rather than better.

Enquire at each follow-up about adverse effects and ask how your patient is getting on with the treatment in general. If adverse effects develop change the dose or the drug.

In elderly patients, or those disabled by arthritis, ensure that the drug is accessible and *not* in a child-proof container.

If it is imperative that a drug be taken but there is serious doubt about patient compliance then slow-release intramuscular depot preparations are available. Examples include phenothiazines, progestogens and iron preparations.

Comment

There is little point in putting a lot of effort and money into reaching a diagnosis if the patient is not going to comply with therapy. The natural history of the underlying disease is then the same as if you had never begun the diagnostic evaluation. Poor compliance should always be borne in mind and efforts made to ensure that treatment is taken as prescribed. Among the various methods for improving compliance the one which is more important than all the others is patient counselling. Explain the reasons for drug therapy clearly to your patient and on subsequent review continue to ask sympathetically about the progress of treatment.

CHAPTER 27

Therapeutic decision making

27.1 The patient

27.2 The doctor

Beware you be not swallowed up in books!
An ounce of love is worth a pound of knowledge.

John Wesley (1703–1791)

Although it is unlikely that Wesley was thinking of therapeutic decision making when he said this, the sentiment is at the very heart of patient management. It is easy to write a prescription, but doing the best for your patient often requires much more effort. The enormous increase in availability of potent pharmacological agents in recent years has in many ways added to the difficulty and complexity of overall patient management. Until the middle of this century the range of possible therapeutic agents was limited, and it was accepted by both the profession and the public that there were many situations in which the doctor could do little more than offer comfort, sympathy and support. Now that we have drugs which can interfere to some extent with virtually every disease process, there is often a feeling among doctors and patients alike that every complaint must have a drug which, if not curative, at least is likely to help. This view is far removed from reality. This chapter outlines the multiple factors that should enter into the decision of an individual doctor to treat an individual patient with a drug.

350

27.1   THE PATIENT

At least five categories of patients can be considered.

Those who can undoubtedly be helped by drug treatment

Examples include those with serious bacterial infections, moderate or severe hypertension, asthma or Parkinson's disease. In these circumstances the doctor is faced with a high degree of diagnostic certainty and overwhelming evidence as to the efficacy of drug treatment. The decision to treat is simple. The nature of that treatment depends on the clinical pharmacology of the drugs.

Those who might be helped by drug treatment

This is a much more difficult area and includes both those occasions where there is diagnostic uncertainty, e.g. recurring central chest pain with normal exercise ECG, and those cases where there is controversy as to the benefits of treatment, e.g. mild hypertension. Here we move very definitely into the area of risk to benefit ratio: the possible benefits of treatment must be weighed against the potential risks associated with drug use. An appropriate decision requires comprehensive assessment of the patient, e.g. identification of other cardiovascular risk factors, together with a detailed knowledge and understanding of the clinical pharmacology of the drugs involved.

Those patients who might be helped either by drugs or by non-pharmacological treatment

For instance, if a person who is obese and mildly hypertensive loses weight, this leads to a reduction in blood pressure. However, drug treatment also lower blood pressure. At present it is uncertain whether lowering a mildly elevated blood pressure substantially lessens a person's overall cardiovascular risk so the doctor is faced not only with the problem of which type of treatment to use, but whether any treatment is indicated.

Those who can be helped—but not by drug therapy

Probably the most common example would be the patient who presents with apparently somatic complaints which have their origins in problems at home or at work. It may be tempting to prescribe a hypnotic for difficulty in sleeping or an antacid for non-specific abdominal pain, but what is often required is time, sympathy and insight to identify the underlying cause.

Those who cannot be helped

It is important in medicine, as in all other aspects of life, to recognise that there is a limit to what one can do. We all encounter patients who for one reason or another simply cannot be helped. This may be because their disease is currently incurable or it may be that they have no identifiable pathology as such but that their problem is immersed in the social and domestic complexities of a lifetime. There is no point in pretending something can be done when the opposite is patently the case. In particular, it does no good for the doctor–patient relationship if hopes of successful treatment are destroyed by experience. An honest opinion is appreciated in the long-term even if it is difficult both to provide and accept in the short term.

27.2 THE DOCTOR

The decision of the doctor whether or not to treat and, if so, with which drug can also be categorised as follows.

Diagnostic certainty and evidence of therapeutic efficacy

If a diagnosis is certain and there is strong evidence that a particular form of drug therapy will be effective then the decision to treat is easy and most doctors would act along very similar lines, with any differences being more in the details rather than in the principles of drug use.

However, when the diagnosis is less certain and there is doubt about the value of drug treatment there is a greater disparity in the approach of different doctors. For example, mild pre-eclampsia in pregnancy is traditionally treated with bed rest, but there is at present no evidence that either bed rest or lowering the blood pressure pharmacologically improves fetal outcome. A survey on the management of pre-eclampsia in the UK showed that older obstetricians tended to use bedrest and tranquillisers. Younger obstetricians tended to use anti-hypertensive drugs. Another example is provided by the Hypertension Detection and Follow-up Program in the USA. 70% of patients treated at specialised centres were still receiving treatment compared to 54% whose treatment was undertaken by non-specialist doctors.

In many instances the decision whether or not to use drug therapy no doubt rests on such evidence as might be available concerning its potential value. In other cases, however, the decision appears also to depend on an individual doctor's willingness to use drugs in general. Thus when patterns of prescribing are viewed on an epidemiological basis it is found that certain doctors are responsible for a disproportionately high number of prescriptions while others are responsible for lower than the average number.

Choice of drug

In an ideal world drug prescribing would be based on a rational and informed assessment of the clinical pharmacology of the agent in question. Regrettably one only has to look at the patterns of prescribing to see that actual practice is very different. All too often a successful marketing campaign may over-ride the benefits of an alternative, possibly cheaper or more effective preparation.

The success of combination tablets of thiazides and potassium sparing agents, which confers no proven benefits over thiazides alone is a good example. One of the most widely prescribed combination preparations costs ten times more per tablet than bendrofluazide, yet is no more effective in controlling hypertension. Such inappropriate drug use is a testament to the success of marketing techniques which aim to imprint the proprietary name of a particular product firmly in the mind of prescribing doctors.

In general terms the use of one preparation rather than another is going to have little, if any, impact on the quality of therapeutic effect. However, the substantial differences in cost to the individual, or the national drug bill, should be borne in mind when choosing a drug. As described in Chapter 24 it is preferable to develop the habit of generic prescribing using approved drug names.

Comment

The factors involved in therapeutic decision making include, but also go far beyond, the principles and practices which have been described in this book, but four general points can be made.

(1) Do not treat until you know what you are treating. Symptomatic treatment may often be justified but should not replace clinical investigation, diagnosis and management of the underlying disease.

(2) Having reached a diagnosis use your knowledge of the likely outcome of the disease, the proven benefits of drug treatment and the proven risks of drug treatment, to decide whether or not you will prescribe a drug.

(3) Having decided to prescribe a drug, choose one which can be conveniently administered.

(4) Recognise and accept the limitations of drug treatment. Advances in clinical pharmacology and our unprecedented ability to put drug treatment on a rational basis in no way undermine the traditional role of the doctor as comforter and friend.

Reference volumes and further reading

Pharmacology

BOWMAN W.C. AND RAND M.J. (1980) *Textbook of Pharmacology*, 2nd Edition. Oxford: Blackwell Scientific Publications.

GILMAN A.G., GOODMAN L.S. AND GILMAN A. eds. (1980) *Goodman and Gilman's The Pharmacological Basis of Therapeutics*, 6th Edition. London: Baillière Tindall.

Medicine

BEESON P.B., MCDERMOTT W. AND WYNGAARDEN J.B. eds. (1979) *Cecil Loeb Textbook of Medicine*, 15th Edition. Philadelphia: Saunders.

MACLEOD J. ed. (1981) *Davidson's Principles and Practice of Medicine*, 13th Edition. Edinburgh: Churchill Livingstone.

WINTROBE M.M. *et al.* eds. (1980) *Harrison's Principles of Internal Medicine*, 9th Edition. New York: McGraw Hill.

Clinical Pharmacology

AVERY G.S. ed. (1980) *Drug Treatment*, 2nd edition. Edinburgh: Churchill Livingstone.

MELMON K.L. AND MORELLI H.F., eds. (1978) *Clinical Pharmacology: basic principles in therapeutics*, 2nd Edition. London: Baillière, Tindall.

356   THERAPEUTIC DECISION MAKING

RICHENS A. AND MARKS V., eds. (1981) *Therapeutic Drug Monitoring*. Edinburgh: Churchill Livingstone.

ROWLAND M. AND TOZER N. (1980) *Clinical Pharmacokinetics: concepts and applications*. Philadelphia: Lea and Febiger.

Other suggested reading

CALMAN K.C., SMYTHE J.F. AND TATTERSALL M.H.N. (1980) *Basic Principles of Cancer Chemotherapy*. London: Macmillan.

CATZEL P. AND OLVER R.E. (1981) *The Paediatric Prescriber*, 5th Edition. Oxford: Blackwell Scientific Publications.

CROOKS J. AND STEVENSON I.H., eds. (1979) *Drugs and the Elderly*. London: Macmillan.

DAVIES D.M. (1977) *Textbook of Adverse Drug Reactions*. Oxford: Oxford University Press.

DUKES M.M.G., ed. (1980) *Meyler's Side Effects of Drugs*, 9th Edition. Amsterdam: Excerpta Medica.

GARROD L.P.M., LAMBERT H.P. AND O'GRADY F. (1980) *Antibiotics and Chemotherapy*, 5th Edition. Edinburgh: Churchill Livingstone.

HANSTEN P.D. (1979) *Drug Interactions*. Philadelphia: Lea and Febiger.

HOLLISTER L.G. (1978) *Clinical Pharmacology of Psychotherapeutic Drugs*. Edinburgh: Churchill Livingstone.

PROUDFOOT A. (1982) *Diagnosis and Management of Acute Poisoning*. Oxford: Blackwell Scientific Publications.

STOCKLEY I.H. (1981) *Drug Interactions: a source book of adverse interactions, their mechanisms, clinical importance and management*. Oxford: Blackwell Scientific Publications.

Index

Bold figures indicate main page reference

357